Good Carbs vs. Bad Carbs

Other Books by the Author

GOOD FAT VS. BAD FAT

THE BIKINI DIET

20/20 THINKING

FOODS THAT COMBAT CANCER

CONTROL DIABETES IN SIX EASY STEPS

WRINKLE-FREE:
YOUR GUIDE TO YOUTHFUL SKIN AT ANY AGE

THE BONE DENSITY TEST

THE CELLULITE BREAKTHROUGH

HAIR SAVERS FOR WOMEN:
A COMPLETE GUIDE TO TREATING AND
PREVENTING HAIR LOSS

NATURAL WEIGHT LOSS MIRACLES

21 DAYS TO BETTER FITNESS

KAVA:
THE ULTIMATE GUIDE TO NATURE'S ANTI-STRESS HERB

Other Books Coauthored by the Author

LEAN BODIES

LEAN BODIES TOTAL FITNESS

30 DAYS TO SWIMSUIT LEAN

HIGH PERFORMANCE NUTRITION

POWER EATING

SHAPE TRAINING

HIGH PERFORMANCE BODYBUILDING

50 WORKOUT SECRETS

BUILT! THE NEW BODYBUILDING FOR EVERYONE

good carbs
vs.
BAD CARBS

Maggie Greenwood-Robinson, Ph.D.

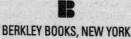

BERKLEY BOOKS, NEW YORK

GOOD CARBS VS. BAD CARBS

A Berkley Book / published by arrangement with the author

PRINTING HISTORY
Berkley edition / January 2004

Copyright © 2004 by Maggie Greenwood-Robinson, Ph.D.
Text design by Kristin del Rosario
Cover design by Rita Frangie

ISBN: 0-425-19384-5

BERKLEY®
Berkley Books are published by The Berkley Publishing Group,
a division of Penguin Group (USA) Inc.,
375 Hudson Street, New York, New York 10014.
BERKLEY and the "B" design
are trademarks belonging to Penguin Group (USA) Inc.

PRINTED IN THE UNITED STATES OF AMERICA

10 9 8 7 6 5 4 3 2 1

To Dad, with love

CONTENTS

ACKNOWLEDGMENTS

Good Carbs vs. Bad Carbs has become a reality due to the effort and energy of the following people: Christina Zika and the staff at Berkley Books; Madeleine Morel, my literary agent; and my husband, Jeff, who has given me the encouragement and support to persevere in my career. To these people, I am very grateful.

I would also like to thank a number of fine organizations that gave me permission to reprint their healthy, delicious carbohydrate recipes: the American Association of Cancer Research, the California Artichoke Advisory Board, the California Avocado Commission, the California Kiwifruit Commission, the Northarvest Bean Growers Association, the Pioneer Valley Growers Association, the U.S. Highbush Blueberry Council, and the U.S. Potato Board. I have included their websites in chapter 12 so you can try some of their many other fabulous recipes.

PART I

Getting to Know
Your Carbohydrates

ONE

The Food Fuel

A big battle has been raging on the diet and nutrition front—the battle between "good" carbohydrates and "bad" carbohydrates. The point of contention has to do with this: Not all carbohydrates are created equal. For instance, there are some that will help prevent all sorts of life-shortening illnesses, from obesity to heart disease to cancer. Still others (like sugar and junk food) can set into motion harmful biochemical reactions inside your body that incite disease.

Obviously, if you want to stay healthy and in terrific shape for as long as you can, you should eat more carbohydrates from the first group and less from the second. And that's exactly what this book helps you do. It helps you discern between foods containing good carbohydrates (natural foods and fiber), which confer enormous health benefits, and bad carbohydrates (sugar, processed foods, and junk carbs), which are less valuable and, in excess quantities or unbalanced dietary proportions, can actually hurt your health and lead to unsightly weight gain.

When you begin to understand the differences among

various types of carbohydrates, you can make better food
choices and enhance your health, lose weight, boost your
physical and mental performance, and protect yourself
against disease or its progression. As you read through
these pages, be prepared for a few startling surprises about
carbs:

- How to boost your brainpower, feel upbeat practically
  all the time, and expand your power of recall—all with
  good carbs.

- A way for you to lose weight permanently and *not* cut
  carbs from your diet. In fact, there are certain carbs
  you must eat if you want to get on the path to lifelong
  slimness and good health.

- Scientific proof that sugar might be more damaging to
  your heart than even fat.

- Ways to feel fully energized to give your body the fat-
  burning boost it needs so you look and feel younger.

- How to plan your meals with a variety of certain types
  of carbs—and live a lot longer.

If you are ready to start living with more control over
your weight and your health than ever before, the information in this book will get you to your goals. With this
in mind, let's get started with a short nutritional lesson on
how carbohydrates, in general, work in your body.

CARBOHYDRATES 101

Whether it is the cereal you had for breakfast or the roll
you ate at dinner, all carbohydrates are organic compounds containing carbon, hydrogen, and oxygen. Carbohydrates are formed directly or indirectly from green

plants through a process called "photosynthesis," which you probably learned about in grade school. In this process, the sun's energy is captured by chlorophyll, the green coloring in leaves, to turn water from the soil and carbon dioxide from the air into an energy-yielding sugar called glucose. Plants require glucose for growth and repair, and any extra, unneeded glucose is converted to starch and stored in the plant.

Carbohydrates are amazingly diverse, present in foods not only as sugars and starch, but also as fiber. Sugars are sometimes called "simple" sugars, a term that describes their chemical structure. Simple sugars, for example, are constructed of either single (monosaccharide) or double (disaccharide) molecules of sugar. The three major single sugars are glucose, fructose, and galactose. Glucose and fructose are found mostly in fruits and vegetables, and galactose is a component of milk and other dairy products.

When two single sugars link up chemically, a double sugar is formed. The most common double sugar is sucrose, better known as table sugar. Sucrose is composed of glucose and fructose and is one of the sweetest of all sugars. Found in sugar cane and sugar beets, sucrose is purified and refined to provide the various sugar products you see on grocery store shelves: table sugar, candy, cakes, cookies, and other sweets.

A pairing of galactose and glucose yields the milk sugar lactose, found in dairy foods. Another double sugar is maltose, which is constructed from two units of glucose. Maltose is found in plants during the early stages of germination. Sugars, regardless of their molecular makeup, are very easily and quickly digested in the body.

Starches are created when three or more glucose molecules hook up. Most plant foods, including cereals, whole grains, pasta, fruits, and vegetables, are starches, also known as complex carbohydrates. Starches take longer to digest than sugars do.

Found in starches and in less-starchy vegetables like lettuce, fiber is the indigestible remnant of plant food. Although it contributes little energy to your diet, fiber provides bulk, which is vital for intestinal action. Fiber has an array of health benefits: It improves elimination, flushes cancer-causing substances from the system, and helps normalize cholesterol levels. A diet high in fiber will help you control your weight, too—in several ways. Fiber makes you feel full so you don't overeat. More energy (calories) is spent digesting and absorbing high-fiber foods. In fact, if you increase your fiber intake to 35 grams a day, you'll automatically burn 250 calories a day, without exercising more or eating less. And fiber helps move food through your system more efficiently. This means fewer calories are left to be stored as fat.

Making up roughly half the calories consumed in the average American diet, carbohydrates are to your body what gas is to your car—the fuel that gets you going. During digestion, all sugars and starches are broken down into glucose (blood sugar) for energy. Assisted by a hormone called insulin, blood glucose is then ushered into cells to be used by various tissues in the body. Carbohydrates, therefore, nourish your body's tissues, providing energy for your brain, central nervous system, and muscle cells in the form of glucose.

Several things can then happen to glucose in your body. Once inside a cell, it can be quickly metabolized to supply energy. Or it might be converted to either liver or muscle glycogen, the storage form of carbohydrate. When you exercise or use your muscles, your body mobilizes muscle glycogen for energy. Blood glucose can also turn into body fat and get packed away in fat tissue. This happens when you eat more carbohydrates than you need or than your body can store as glycogen. Some blood glucose might also be excreted in your urine.

Above all other nutrients, your body prefers to run on

glucose from carbohydrates, even though two other nutrients, fat and protein, can provide energy, too. Fat is considered a food fuel, but it is more of an understudy or backup source. Only if carbohydrate stores dwindle will your body tap in to fat for fuel.

Protein is not a good source of energy for your body and is, in fact, underemployed when called upon as an energy provider. Its most important job in your body is to build and repair tissue. Using protein as an energy source is like hiring a computer specialist, then relegating him to the mailroom. Protein simply has more important jobs to do in the body than supply energy.

If you don't eat enough carbohydrates or fat, however, protein will be used as an energy source, because energy production takes metabolic priority over tissue-building. But the problem is that food protein and body protein (muscle and other tissue) will be sacrificed to supply energy, causing parts of your body to waste away. So you see, carbs hold fort as your body's best supply of energy.

MEET THE CARBOHYDRATE FOODS

*Getting familiar with the foods that supply the carbo*hydrates your body needs is the first essential step toward making healthier food choices. Here is an overview of the main carbohydrate food categories.

Grains and Cereals

Since ancient times, grains and cereals have been considered vital to life, signifying their remarkable nutritional value. They are "near-complete" foods because they contain protein, carbohydrates, and beneficial fats.

But the benefits don't stop there. Grains are loaded with a slew of trace minerals, including blood-building iron.

Grains keep cholesterol levels in check; exert a cancer-protective effect on the body, particularly on the digestive system; contain blood-pressure-lowering nutrients such as potassium; and are packed with B vitamins, which are involved in metabolism (your body's food-to-fuel process).

Grains and cereals come from grasses that yield edible seeds. The most commonly cultivated grains are wheat, rice, rye, oats, barley, corn, and sorghum. Generally, these are available in their raw grain form or as ingredients in other foods such as breads and prepared cereals.

One of the oldest cultivated plants is wheat, the most widely grown grain today. Wheat is used to produce breakfast cereals and flour for various types of bakery products and pastas. In its unprocessed form, wheat is high in B vitamins and fiber. However, the milling process that refines wheat into various commercial forms removes the wheat bran and wheat germ, where the beneficial nutrients are most plentiful.

The second largest grain crop in the world is rice, a staple of all Asian countries. Unlike wheat, which is grown on large farms and cultivated mechanically, rice is grown on small paddies (fields that are submerged in water) and harvested by hand. Rice is a popular food on its own and available in many varieties. It is also used in breakfast cereals and to make alcoholic beverages such as sake. Rice that has been processed to remove only the husks is known as brown rice. It is rich in calcium, iron, and several B vitamins. White rice has been milled to remove the bran and, thus, contains fewer nutrients.

Originating in southwestern Asia around 6500 B.C.E., rye is used mostly in bread and other bakery products, as well as in distilled liquors. Nutritionally, rye supplies small amounts of potassium and B vitamins. Most of the world's rye is now grown in Poland.

A very popular grain is oat, widely available in break-

fast cereals and some breads. The oatmeal you eat for
breakfast is actually the flattened kernel of the oat seed
with the hulls removed. Another derivative of the grain,
oat flour, is used in cookies and puddings. Highly nutritious, oat grains also contain protein and fat. They are an
excellent source of calcium and iron, as well as various
B vitamins.

Barley is among the most ancient of grains, dating back
to 5000 B.C.E. in Egypt. It was the chief grain of the
Hebrews, Greeks, and Romans through the sixteenth cen-
tury. Among the most nutritious forms of barley is pearled
barley, made of whole kernels from which the outer husk
and part of the bran have been removed. Barley supplies
the malt used in the brewing of beer and the distillation
of liquor. It is also an ingredient in various breakfast
foods. Barley is high in calcium and phosphorus.

Originally cultivated by Indians in the Americas, corn
was later introduced to Europe by Columbus and other
explorers. There are many different varieties of corn, including yellow, white, red, blue, pink, and black. Corn is
eaten as a fresh, canned, or frozen food and is widely used
in other foods, including popcorn, tortillas, and various
bakery products. In nutritional value, however, corn is in-
ferior to other grains, lacking in protein and the B vitamin
niacin.

Although principally an animal feed, sorghum is used
to make a sweet syrup for cooking and baking. In many
countries around the world, it is ground into a meal that
can be made into porridge, flatbreads, and cakes.

There are also various specialty grains that have gained
favor over the years for their high nutritional value. One
of these is quinoa (*KEEN-wa*), which is technically an
herb, although it looks like a grain. Quinoa, available in
breakfast cereals, is unusual in that it is supremely high
in protein. Unlike most grains, it contains all nine essential amino acids, the vital protein components of food.

Other specialty grains include kasha (buckwheat groats), which can be used as a side dish or a meat substitute; and couscous, a popular Mideastern grain.

Starchy Vegetables

Foods in this category include potatoes, sweet potatoes, yams, beets, and winter squash. These foods are brimming with vitamins, minerals, fiber, and health-building plant chemicals.

Yellow or orange starchy vegetables are particularly healthful. They contain beneficial plant chemicals called carotenoids such as beta-carotene that have "provitamin A activity," meaning that your body produces vitamin A from them. They also protect your cells against damage that could lead to health problems. With their many nutritional "pluses," starchy vegetables are an important component of a healthy diet.

Peas and Legumes

These energy-loaded foods include black beans, black-eyed chickpeas (garbanzos), kidney beans, lentils, lima beans, navy beans, pinto beans, soybeans, split peas, white beans, and even peanuts.

There are 13,000 kinds of legumes, but only about twenty are used as food by humans. Among those twenty, there is a wide variety of colors, sizes, shapes, and flavors. Calorie-wise though, most dry beans are similar. A half-cup serving provides between 110 and 143 calories of energy-giving carbohydrates.

Some legumes, such as soybeans and peanuts, are cultivated for both their protein and their oil content. Others, like lentils, lima beans, chickpeas, and peas, are grown for their value as protein sources. In either case, these foods are among the most nourishing of all vegetables—

and are extremely high in fiber. Beans are also packed with vitamins, especially thiamin, riboflavin, niacin, and folate; and minerals, including calcium, iron, copper, zinc, phosphorus, potassium, and magnesium.

Fruits and Vegetables

Fruits and certain vegetables other than legumes are not as high in starch as other carbohydrate foods, but they are loaded with other vital nutrients that protect your body against disease. These include vitamins, minerals, antioxidants, and a variety of natural plant chemicals called "phytochemicals" that have wide-ranging health benefits. All these nutrients are known to guard against cancer, heart disease, and other life-threatening illnesses. Eating a fruit- and vegetable-based diet ensures that you get the greatest variety of disease-fighting nutrients.

An easy way to do that is to make it a habit to eat one or more servings a day from each of these categories of fruits and vegetables: citrus fruits; noncitrus fruits, including berries; green and dark-green leafy vegetables, including spinach and romaine lettuce; yellow/orange or red vegetables such as sweet peppers, carrots, and squash; and "cruciferous" vegetables such as broccoli, Brussels sprouts, or cabbage. Cruciferous vegetables are so named because their reproductive structures contain components that are arranged like a cross, hence the name "cruciferous," which comes from a word meaning "to place on a cross," or "crucify."

Dairy Products

You probably don't think of dairy products as carbohydrates, but these foods do hold an appreciable amount of the nutrient. Most dairy products contain lactose, the only major carbohydrate other than galactose that comes from an animal source. Lactose is important because it stimulates the absorption of calcium from your intestine.

Some people, however, are sensitive to lactose—a condition called "lactose intolerance"—because they lack sufficient lactase, the enzyme required to digest lactose. If you are lactose intolerant, you can't drink milk without getting an upset stomach. If you have problems digesting milk, try using lactase enzyme replacers, such as Lactaid or Dairyease, which can help you add more milk to your diet, or include yogurt in your diet. Yogurt is more easily digested if you're lactose intolerant. Check the label to make sure it contains live active yogurt cultures such as *L. acidophilus*, which can destroy dangerous food-borne bacteria and, thus, offer protection against disease.

Sugars, Natural and Added

Sugar in our diets comes in two forms: naturally occurring sugar and added sugar, or what scientists called "extrinsic sugar." Naturally occurring sugar is found in fruits and vegetables, dairy products, and such sources as sugar cane, sugar beets, and honey. Virtually all the calories supplied by fruit come in the form of sugar.

The most common form of added sugar is what you know as table sugar, which is incorporated into food, baked goods, desserts, candies and sweets, and processed foods. Another type of added sugar is "high-fructose corn syrup," a refined version of fructose made from cornstarch and found in soft drinks, beverages, and many processed foods. You'll learn more about high-fructose corn syrup and other added sugars in the next chapter.

The amount of added sugar in the American diet is on the rise. In 1970, we ate about 120 pounds of sugar per year; today, we eat 150 pounds a year, or almost a half-pound a day. Most of this sugar comes from the soft drinks we consume, as well as from table sugar, jams, and syrups.

Alcohol

Considered a minor carbohydrate, alcohol is formed during a process called fermentation in which sugars and starches are broken down by yeast. Beer, for example, is made by fermenting barley and hops; wine, by fermenting grapes and other fruits; and hard liquor, by fermenting various grains or potatoes. After fermentation, the liquid is distilled to concentrate the alcohol.

Your body uses alcohol as an energy source, but it is not converted to glucose as other carbohydrates are. Instead, it is converted into fatty acids (components of fat). When consumed in excess of what is burned off, alcohol will be turned into fat and stored.

Alcohol provides nothing more than calories to your diet; it contains no protein and very few vitamins or minerals. Although there are some beneficial plant chemicals in beer and wine, you can obtain the very same substances from fruits and vegetables. From a nutritional perspective, alcohol cannot be recommended as a component of a balanced diet and should be used in moderation, if at all.

AN ENERGIZING NUTRIENT

Clearly, carbohydrates are a vital nutrient for good health, supplying the get-up-and-go you need to get up and go, plus providing a bounty of vitamins, minerals, fiber, and other protective nutrients. They are the mainstay of a good diet, provided you learn how to select the healthiest carbs possible. That's where we are headed in the next chapter.

TWO

Carbohydrate Scorecards

Carbs are the "enemy" nutrient of the moment, but what is the real story anyway? What carbs should you eat, and what carbs should you avoid? Let's start answering these questions by decoding carbohydrates so you can see which ones work for you nutritionally (the good carbs) and which ones work against you (the bad carbs).

There are essentially three ways to grade carbohydrates to figure out which ones yield the most bang for your nutritional buck. The carbohydrate "scorecards" are as follows:

- Simple versus complex

- Fast versus slow

- Low fiber versus high fiber

Each of these appraisal systems has its pluses and minuses, so it's best to become familiar with all three methods. When you begin to look at carbs from all three dimensions, you will have a sharper understanding of which ones best suit your individual health requirements. Then, you can begin to customize your diet to accommodate your body's true carbohydrate needs. Right now, the carbohydrate picture might look a little fuzzy to you, but trust me, it will come into much sharper focus by the time you finish this chapter.

SCORECARD #1: SIMPLE VERSUS COMPLEX

Carbohydrates are traditionally categorized as either simple or *complex*, a classification that is based on the molecular structure of the carbohydrate, with simple carbohydrates, or sugars, constructed of either single or double molecules of sugar, and complex carbohydrates (starches) made of multiple numbers of sugar molecules. As I pointed out in the previous chapter, simple sugars are found in table sugar, jams, candies, syrups, and processed foods; complex carbohydrates are found in whole grains, cereals, beans, fruits, and vegetables.

The value of grading carbohydrates in terms of simple versus complex lies in the ability to assess their overall nutrient value. If you desire the highest possible nutrition in your diet, you would choose mostly complex carbohydrates, for example. These foods are packed with nutrients, including dietary fiber, which has a long list of impressive health benefits. Fruits and vegetables, in particular, supply vitamins and minerals, two classes of nutrients vital to health. Several vitamins and minerals, namely beta-carotene, vitamin C, vitamin E, and the mineral selenium, are known as "antioxidants." At the cellular level, antioxidants sweep up disease-causing substances known as "free radicals." Free radicals are volatile toxic molecules that cause harmful reactions in the body. In some cases, free radicals puncture cell membranes, preventing the intake of nutrients and, thus, starving the cells.

In others, they tinker with the body's genetic material. This produces mutations that cause cells to act abnormally and reproduce uncontrollably. Dreaded diseases like cancer are often the result. In addition to cancer, scientists have linked some sixty diseases to free radicals, among them: heart disease, Alzheimer's disease, and arthritis. Antioxidants guard against free radical damage and are, thus, health-protective. An antioxidant-rich diet—one plentiful in complex carbohydrates—affords significant health protection against these diseases.

By eating lots of antioxidant-rich complex carbs, you're automatically filling up on another set of nutrients called "phytochemicals," which means "plant chemicals." Neither vitamins nor minerals, phytochemicals occur naturally in all fruits, vegetables, and grains. They exert their health-protecting action by various biochemical mechanisms, and the results are nothing short of amazing. Phytochemicals appear to protect against cancer, heart disease, and many other life-threatening illnesses. With their wealth of antioxidants and phytochemicals, you can certainly score complex carbohydrates "good carbs."

Simple carbohydrates, by contrast, are generally lacking in vitamins, minerals, antioxidants, and phytochemicals. Most of the food we commonly describe as "junk food" falls in the simple carbohydrate category. These foods supply a lot of calories but very little in the way of good nutrition. Thus, if your diet is overly high in simple carbohydrates, you're at risk for nutritional deficiencies. By that token, simple carbohydrates can be graded as "bad carbs." For an overview of complex and simple carbohydrates, see the following table.

Who Should Use Scorecard #1?

Answer: everyone. Evaluating carbs as to whether they are simple or complex is the easiest way to make healthy food choices. This scorecard works universally—for weight control, disease prevention and management, and all-around healthy eating.

	EAT MORE OF THESE:	EAT LESS OF THESE:
	Complex Carbohydrates (Good Carbs)	*Simple Carbohydrates (Bad Carbs)*
Beverages	Freshly squeezed juice Natural juices, no sugar added	Alcoholic beverages Any sugared drink Flavored coffees and teas Fruit punches Juice drinks, sugar added Lemonades Punches Sugared soft drinks Sugared waters
Bread, Grain, and Cereal Products	Whole-grain breads Whole grains and cereals	Cakes, cookies, other baked goods Crackers, chips, and other snack foods (potato chips, taco chips, corn chips, pretzels, cheese curls, etc.) Croissants, muffins, and biscuits Fried starches (tortillas and taco shells) High-calorie convenience foods Pies Pizza dough Presweetened cereals Sweet breads White breads and rolls White pastas White rice

(continued)

	EAT MORE OF THESE:	EAT LESS OF THESE:
	Complex Carbohydrates (Good Carbs)	*Simple Carbohydrates (Bad Carbs)*
Dairy Products	Fat-free milk Low-fat milk Skim milk Yogurt, sugar free	Chocolate milk Frozen desserts Ice cream Ice milk Milk shakes Puddings, sugar added Soft ice cream Whole milk Yogurt, sugar added
Fruits	Fresh fruits Frozen fruits, no added sugar Fruits canned in their own juice or packed in water	Fruits canned in syrup Fruits to which sugar has been added
Vegetables	Canned vegetables, no added sugar or fat Frozen vegetables, no added sugar or fat Legumes Lightly cooked vegetables Raw vegetables	French fries Instant mashed potatoes Vegetables with added sugar Vegetables with cream sauces

SCORECARD #2: FAST VERSUS SLOW

This grading system ranks carbohydrates by how they affect your blood sugar levels. Technically, this system is termed the "glycemic index," and it was invented in the early 1980s by researchers at the University of Toronto. Essentially, the glycemic index is a scale describing how fast a food is converted to glucose in your blood. Foods on the index are rated numerically, with glucose at 100.

The higher the number assigned to a food, the faster it converts to glucose. Foods with a rating of 70 or higher are generally considered high-glycemic index foods (high-GI foods); a rating of 55 to 69, moderate-glycemic index foods (moderate-GI foods); and below 55, low-glycemic index foods (low-GI foods).

High-GI foods tend to cause a rapid surge of insulin (the hormone that helps usher glucose into cells for fuel), followed by a plunge of blood sugar that can lead to low energy. By contrast, low-GI foods produce a slow, steady release of insulin and yield more sustained energy. Theoretically, you can use the index to select carbohydrates that are less likely to cause roller-coaster swings in your blood sugar.

Why is this important? Whether a carbohydrate causes a fast release (high-GI carbs) or a slow release (low-GI carbs) can have dramatic effects on many aspects of your health—all due to insulin and its effects on your body. At normal levels, insulin is a vital hormone, with many important functions in the body. But when repeatedly elevated, insulin is harmful, contributing to diabetes, obesity, heart disease, and possibly cancer.

In diabetes, for example, the glycemic index can help patients select foods that help them better control their blood sugar. Research shows that a low-GI diet lowers blood glucose and insulin levels significantly compared to diets of high-GI foods. Scientists also believe that following mostly a low-GI diet might help prevent diabetes.

Low-GI diets might help you control your weight, too. Remember that in response to high-GI foods, insulin spikes upward. This insulin overload activates fat cell enzymes. These enzymes move fat from the bloodstream into fat cells for storage and trigger your body to create more fat cells. High-GI foods thus create conditions in your body that are conducive to gaining fat.

High-GI foods also stimulate your appetite. These carbs

initiate a steep rise in blood sugar, which then drops to subnormal levels about an hour or two after you eat that high-GI meal. This abnormally low level of blood sugar creates a state of hunger. What all this tells us is very simple: High-GI foods promote fat storage; low-GI foods do not. Choosing low-GI carbohydrates makes it possible to lose weight more easily by controlling insulin, fat storage, and your appetite.

Where heart disease is concerned, high levels of insulin can be damaging to your heart. Chronically elevated insulin triggers high blood sugar, elevates triglycerides (a type of blood fat associated with heart disease), and reduces levels of a beneficial type of cholesterol known as HDL.

Then there is the cancer issue. An emerging body of medical research indicates that a high-GI diet might be linked to colon cancer, the third leading cause of disease-related death in the United States. Again, insulin is the villain; it appears to accelerate the development of colon cancer by increasing certain growth factors that lead to uncontrolled cell division.

Now for some caveats: Remember my mentioning that each carbohydrate grading system has its inherent flaws? The glycemic index, despite its usefulness, has a few chinks in its evaluative armor. Here's why: Using the glycemic index to select foods can sometimes be misleading—for at least three reasons. First of all, meals do not consist of single foods. Normally, you eat mixed meals containing protein, carbohydrates, fiber, and some fat.

Mixed meals, thanks to their combination of protein, fiber, and fat, slow your digestion, providing a steady insulin release and, therefore, lowering the glycemic index of the entire meal. The point is, a food's rating on the index does not make much difference as long as it is eaten in slow-release food combinations.

The second problem with this method of rating foods

is that some people choose foods low on the index. Many of these foods are simply not good for you, especially if you're trying to control your weight. Take ice cream, for example. It is a low-glycemic index food because it contains protein and fat, along with high-glycemic sucrose (sugar). Thus, it is broken down very slowly. Although it has a low glycemic index, it is chock-full of fat and sugar. Some foods with a low glycemic index can lead to unwanted body fat and other health problems.

On the other hand, potatoes, cantaloupe, tropical fruits, and pumpkin have a relatively high glycemic index, yet are highly nutritious—good carbs, really. If you shunned such foods, you'd be missing out on foods loaded with vitamins, minerals, and fiber. Letting the glycemic index totally dictate the carbohydrates you choose is not always wise.

The third problem with using the glycemic index is that the ratings of foods can change, depending on their individual characteristics as well as how they are prepared. Take a banana, for example. Its rating practically doubles with its ripeness! In addition, cooking starchy vegetables breaks down their cell walls—a process that increases their glycemic score.

Who Should Use This Scorecard?

The glycemic index remains controversial, and not everyone needs to use it. Judging carbs on whether they are complex or simple works best for most people. Still, there is value in using the glycemic index—in certain cases. Consider using this scorecard if you need to:

- Control your blood sugar, particularly if you have diabetes or want to prevent it, especially if it runs in your family.
- Watch your weight.

* Tame an out-of-control appetite (in research, low-glycemic foods have been deemed more filling than high-glycemic foods).

* Control levels of certain blood fats (see chapter 8 for more information).

The glycemic index is also useful in sports nutrition. Low-glycemic foods eaten prior to long bouts of exercise have been found to extend endurance time. High-glycemic index foods eaten after exercise are more effective at rapidly restoring carbohydrates lost from muscles as a result of training or working out.

In the following tables, you'll find the glycemic index of some common carbohydrate foods.

LOW-GLYCEMIC INDEX CARBOHYDRATES (LESS THAN 55)

Beverages	*Whole milk	27
	Soy milk	31
	Fat-free milk	32
	Skim milk	32
	*Chocolate milk	34
	Apple juice	41
	Carrot juice	45
	Pineapple juice	46
	Grapefruit juice	48
	Cranberry juice cocktail	52
Bread, Grain, and Cereal Products	Pearled barley	25
	Fettuccine	32
	Whole-wheat spaghetti	37
	Spaghetti	41
	Pumpernickel bread	41
	All-bran cereal	42
	Macaroni	45
	Bulgur wheat	46

(continued)

LOW-GLYCEMIC INDEX CARBOHYDRATES (LESS THAN 55)

Bread, Grain, and Cereal Products	Banana bread	47
	Long-grain rice	47
	Parboiled rice	47
	Old-fashioned oatmeal	49
	Oat bran	50
	Stone-ground, whole-wheat bread	53
	Special K cereal	54
Dairy Products	Low-fat, sugar-free yogurt	14
	Low-fat with sugar yogurt	33
	Low-fat ice cream	50
Fruits	Berries	15
	Cherries	22
	Plums	24
	Grapefruit	25
	Peaches	28
	Canned peaches	30
	Banana, underripe	30
	Dried apricots	31
	Apples	36
	Pears	36
	Grapes	43
	Oranges	43
	Kiwifruit	52
	Bananas, ripe	53
Legumes	Peanuts	14
	Soybeans	18
	Kidney beans	27
	Lentils	29
	Black beans	30
	Lima beans	32
	Split peas	32
	Chickpeas	33
	Lentil soup	44
	Pinto beans	45
	Baked beans	48

(continued)

LOW-GLYCEMIC INDEX CARBOHYDRATES (LESS THAN 55)

Vegetables	Tomato soup	38
	Peas	48
	Yams	51
	Sweet potatoes	54
Miscellaneous	Fructose	23
	Candy bars	41
	Potato chips	54
	Oatmeal cookies	54

Eat these foods sparingly. Although low on the glycemic index, they are high in empty calories and provide few nutrients; some of these foods are high in fat.

MODERATE-GLYCEMIC INDEX CARBOHYDRATES (55 TO 69)

Beverages	Orange juice from concentrate	57
	Carbonated soft drinks	68
Bread, Grain, and Cereal Products	Brown rice	55
	Linguine	55
	Popcorn	55
	Sweet corn	55
	White rice	56
	Pita bread	57
	Mini shredded wheat	58
	Blueberry muffins	59
	Bran muffins	60
	Hamburger buns	61
	Granola bars, chewy	61
	Couscous	63
	Instant oatmeal	66

(continued)

MODERATE-GLYCEMIC INDEX CARBOHYDRATES (55 TO 69)

Bread, Grain, and Cereal Products	Grape nuts	67
	Croissants	67
	American rye bread	68
	Taco shells	68
	Whole-wheat bread	69
	Cornmeal	69
Dairy Products	*Ice cream*	61
Fruits	Fruit cocktail, canned	55
	Mangoes	55
	Peaches, canned, heavy syrup	58
	Papayas	58
	Apricots, canned, light syrup	64
	Raisins	64
	Pineapples	66
Legumes	Black bean soup	64
	Green pea soup	66
Vegetables	Beets	64
Miscellaneous	*Table sugar*	65

Eat these foods sparingly. Although relatively low on the glycemic index, they are high in empty calories and provide few nutrients; some of these foods are high in fat.

HIGH-GLYCEMIC INDEX CARBOHYDRATES (70 OR HIGHER)

Beverages	Gatorade	91
Bread, Grain, and Cereal Products	Melba toast	70
	White bread	70
	Bagels	72
	Kaiser rolls	73
	Bran flakes	74
	Cheerios	74
	Cream of wheat, instant	74
	Graham crackers	74
	Saltines	74
	Doughnuts	75
	Frozen waffles	76
	*Total cereal	76
	English muffins	77
	Rice cakes	82
	Rice Krispies	82
	Cornflakes	84
	Rice Chex	89
	Rice, instant	91
	French bread	95
Fruits	*Watermelons	72
Vegetables	*Carrots	71
	*Rutabaga	72
	*Potatoes	85
	*Parsnips	95
Miscellaneous	Corn chips	72
	Honey	73
	Pretzels	83

*Although high on the glycemic index, these are very healthy foods and should not be avoided or limited in your diet.

SCORECARD #3:
LOW FIBER VERSUS HIGH FIBER

*I'm sure you know all about fiber. It's what your grand-*mother used to call "roughage," and what we know as the stuff in fruits, vegetables, and whole grains that keeps us regular. The "push" response of your intestines depends on adequate fiber in your diet. Low amounts of fiber in the diet are linked to dozens of medical problems, including heart disease, some cancers, diabetes, diverticulosis, and gallstones. See the following table for a list.

CONDITIONS AND DISEASES ASSOCIATED WITH POOR DIETARY
FIBER INTAKE

Appendicitis	Gallstones
Cardiovascular disease	Gum disease
Breast cancer	Hemorrhoids
Cholecystitis (inflammation of the gallbladder)	Hiatal hernias
	High blood pressure
Colorectal cancer	High cholesterol
Constipation	Ischemic heart disease
Coronary blood clotting	Kidney stones
Dental cavities	Obesity
Duodenal ulcers	Pyelonephritis (inflammation of the kidney)
Diabetes	Stomach cancer
Diverticulosis	Varicose veins

Just so you know what carbs to avoid: Low-fiber carbs include such foods as white bread, white rice, cream of

wheat, corn flakes, iceberg lettuce, and any simple carbohydrate such as those listed earlier. The more processed
and sugary a food is, the less fiber it contains.

Fiber is essential if you want to stay healthy and active
as long as possible, so it is important to judge carbohydrates in terms of their fiber content. Generally, food labels will help you make this determination. A food is
considered a high-fiber food if it contains at least 2.5 to
3.0 grams of fiber per serving. Without question, high-
fiber foods are considered to be good carbs. In the following table, you'll find a list of some of the best.

HIGH-FIBER FOODS

	Food	Serving Size	Fiber Content (gm)
Beans and Legumes	Beans, kidney, red, canned	½ cup	8
	Peas, split, boiled	½ cup	8
	Lentils, boiled	½ cup	8
	Beans, black, boiled	½ cup	7.5
	Beans, pinto, boiled	½ cup	7.5
	Refried beans, canned	½ cup	6.5
	Lima beans, boiled	½ cup	6.5
	Beans, kidney, red, boiled	½ cup	6.5
	Beans, baked, canned, plain or vegetarian	½ cup	6.5
	Beans, white, canned	½ cup	6.5
Vegetables	Artichokes, boiled	1 cup	9
	Peas, boiled	1 cup	9
	Vegetables, mixed, boiled	1 cup	8
	Lettuce, iceberg	1 head	7.5
	Pumpkin, canned	1 cup	7
	Peas, canned	1 cup	7
	Brussels sprouts, frozen, boiled	1 cup	6
	Parsnips, boiled	1 cup	6
	Sauerkraut, canned	1 cup	6

(continued)

HIGH-FIBER FOODS

	Food	Serving Size	Fiber Content (gm)
Breads, Grains, and Cereals	Fiber One (General Mills)	½ cup	14
	Granola, homemade	½ cup	13
	All-Bran with Extra Fiber (Kellogg's)	½ cup	13
	All-Bran (Kellogg's)	½ cup	9.7
	Bulgur wheat, cooked	½ cup	8
	Raisin Bran (Post)	1 cup	8
	100% Bran (Post)	⅓ cup	8
	Bran Chex (Kellogg's)	1 cup	8
	Shredded wheat and bran	1¼ cup	8
	Oat bran, cooked	½ cup	6
Fruits	Avocadoes, Florida	1 avocado	18
	Raspberries, frozen, unsweetened	1 cup	17
	Prunes, stewed	1 cup	16
	Dates, chopped	1 cup	13
	Pears, dried	10 each	13
	Avocadoes, California	1 avocado	8.7
	Raspberries, raw	1 cup	8
	Blueberries, raw	1 cup	7.6
	Papayas, whole	1 fruit	5.5
	Figs, dried	2 figs	4.6
	Pears	1 medium	3

Source: Nutrient Data Laboratory. USDA Nutrient Database for Standard Reference, Release 14. Beltsville, Maryland.

There are two general types of fiber in foods: soluble and insoluble. Soluble fiber—beta-glucans in oatmeal, pectin in apples, and hemicellulose in beans—dissolves in the presence of water, forming a gummy gel. It is this gel that binds to toxic substances to usher them out of your body. Hemicellulose, in particular, helps lower the amount of fat that is absorbed during digestion. Soluble fiber is also food for the billions of helpful bacteria that reside in your intestines. Good sources of soluble fibers include barley, rice, corn, oats, legumes, apples and pears (especially the fleshy portions), citrus fruits, bananas, carrots, prunes, cranberries, seeds, and seaweed.

Insoluble fiber, which includes lignins, cellulose, and some hemicelluloses, swells in water but does not dissolve in it. Lignins usher bile acids and cholesterol out of the intestines. Cellulose, the roughage we tend to associate with fiber, acts like a stool softener and bulk former, improving elimination and flushing carcinogens from your body. Hemicelluloses do their part by absorbing water in the digestive tract and moving food faster through your system. These actions help relieve constipation, rid the body of cancer-causing substances, and assist in weight control. Good food sources of insoluble fibers include root and leafy vegetables, wheat bran, whole grains (such as wheat, barley, rice, corn, and oats), legumes, unpeeled apples and pears, and strawberries. High-fiber cereals are usually fortified with insoluble fiber.

Fiber Requirements

How much fiber should you eat to get its protective benefits? The current recommendation is 25 to 35 grams of fiber a day from both soluble and insoluble fiber. Most Americans get only about 11 grams a day, however. If you're fiber-needy, try to increase your intake gradually. Doing so can help prevent cramping, bloating, and other unpleasant symptoms often associated with increased fiber. Always drink plenty of water, too—about 8 to 10 glasses of pure water daily—because a high-fiber diet is virtually worthless unless there's enough water in your system to help move the food and fiber through. There are many ways you can sneak fiber into your diet to increase your daily intake, and you will learn about them in this book.

Who Should Use This Scorecard?

Because everyone needs to eat more fiber, everyone can benefit from using this scorecard. Knowing the fiber content of foods and increasing your intake is very important if you need to:

* Manage digestive diseases such as diverticulosis, or prevent constipation.

* Control your weight, as fiber is a top-drawer nutrient for reducing body fat.

* Prevent or treat heart disease or diabetes.

* Protect yourself against cancer and other diseases.

THE SCOOP ON SUGAR

Among simple carbohydrates, sugar, or sucrose, is one of the least desirable carbs to include in your diet. Sugar is unfortunately a major source of calories in the diet, but it is a highly refined food that offers no nutrients to go along with the calories. For this reason, dietitians describe sugar as having "empty calories." Therefore, it's best to restrict it in your diet. Too much sugar has been associated with tooth decay, obesity, cardiovascular disease, cancer, and blood-sugar-metabolism disorders such as diabetes and hypoglycemia (low blood sugar). Unfortunately, sugar and other natural sweeteners are added to a dizzying array of foods, but if you stick to natural, unprocessed carbohydrates, you'll automatically slash your intake of added sugar and never go overboard.

High-Fructose Corn Syrup:
The Sugar That Acts Like a Fat

One particularly troublesome form of added sugar is high-fructose corn syrup. From soft drinks to cereals to energy bars, foods that you probably eat every day are sweetened with this additive, and it might just be the baddest of the bad carbs.

Made from cornstarch, high-fructose corn syrup is a liquid that is predominantly fructose but has some glucose in it. (Even the powdered fructose sold in stores is made from cornstarch and not from refining the sugar in fruit, as you might assume.) Food manufacturers love high-fructose corn syrup because it tastes much sweeter than sugar; this means they can use less of it and save on their manufacturing costs. Consumption of high-fructose corn syrup has risen more than 21 percent since 1970, when it was introduced into the food supply.

Back then, no one knew that it harbored a secret: High-fructose corn syrup is metabolized differently in the body than regular, good ol' sugar. To help you understand these differences, here's a snapshot of what happens:

When you eat sugar, it is rapidly digested and released into your bloodstream, elevating your blood sugar. This triggers the production of insulin by your pancreas to clear the sugar from your blood and into cells to be used for fuel. Besides insulin, sugar also increases the production of leptin, a hormone that acts like an appetite suppressant. Sugar suppresses the secretion of another hormone, ghrelin. Produced mostly by cells in your stomach, ghrelin triggers your desire to eat. So to a certain extent, eating carbohydrates that contain some glucose helps dampen your hunger.

The metabolism of fructose takes an entirely different course. Surprisingly, fructose appears to act more like a fat in the body: It does not trigger insulin production. It does not increase leptin production. Nor does it suppress the production of ghrelin.

Further, if not used first as energy, fructose bypasses a dietary control point that other sugars go through and instead heads directly to your liver, where it is metabolized into triglycerides, a fat. What all this suggests is that eating a lot of fructose, like eating too much fat, might make you gain weight.

Not surprisingly, many scientists believe that fructose, particularly high-fructose corn syrup because it is so prevalent in foods, is a contributing factor to the obesity epidemic in this country. Its increasing consumption has paralleled the rise in obesity among Americans. According to a U.S. Department of Agriculture analysis, from 1985 to 2000, Americans added roughly 330 calories to their daily intake, and 25 percent (about 83 calories) came from sweeteners, including high-fructose corn syrup. That amount of added sugar in your diet will produce a weight gain of nearly nine pounds a year.

Fructose has another downside: Some people suffer from a condition called "fructose intolerance"—a sensitivity to the fructose in fruit juices, sports drinks, or products containing high-fructose corn syrup, and sometimes to the natural fructose in fruit. Symptoms include stomach upset, diarrhea, and bloating. In rare cases in which someone lacks the enzyme needed to digest fructose, the symptoms will be more severe: vomiting, hypoglycemia (low blood sugar), jaundice, or enlarged liver. You can be tested for fructose intolerance with a breath test or a blood test. If diagnosed with this condition, you'll have to avoid foods containing fructose, especially high-fructose corn syrup.

Another fructose alert: Research with fructose has discovered that high levels of fructose in the diet can keep the body from properly using magnesium and copper, two essential minerals.

Hidden Sugars

Go on alert that you might be eating more sugar than you think you are due to hidden sugars and sweeteners. A food could still contain simple sugars but under the guise of names like honey, molasses, corn syrup, and, yes, high-fructose corn syrup. The World Health Organization (WHO) now recommends that you limit your intake of added sugars to 10 percent of your total daily calories. So if you eat 2,000 calories daily, this works out to 200 calories, the amount found in a slice of apple pie, a half-cup of ice cream, or a can and a half of cola.

In the accompanying table, you will find many of the different forms of sugars found in food. If these ingredients appear first or second on a label's list of ingredients, the product is too high in added sugars. Be a wise consumer. Make sure you know what you're buying—and what you're eating.

HIDDEN SUGARS IN YOUR FOOD

Sugar (sucrose)	Refined crystallized sap of the sugar cane or sugar beet; a combination of glucose and fructose.
Dextrose (glucose)	Another name for glucose. A simple sugar that is less sweet than fructose or sucrose.
Lactose	A simple sugar from milk; less sweet than sucrose, fructose, or maltose.
Maltose	A simple sugar made from starch; less sweet than sucrose or fructose.
Maltodextrin	A manufactured sugar from maltose and dextrose in corn.
Brown sugar	A refined sugar coated with molasses. The minerals calcium, iron, and potassium are present in this sugar.

(continued)

HIDDEN SUGARS IN YOUR FOOD

Raw Sugar	A less-refined sugar that still has some natural molasses coating.
Fructose	A simple sugar refined from fruit.
Molasses	The syrup separated from sugar crystals during the refining process. Blackstrap molasses, a popular health food, is a good source of calcium, iron, and potassium.
Honey	A concentrated solution of fructose and glucose (80 percent) and some sucrose. Produced by bees from the nectar of flowers.
Maple syrup	A concentrated sap from sugar maple trees, predominantly fructose.
Corn syrup	A manufactured syrup of cornstarch, containing varying proportions of glucose, maltose, and dextrose.
High-fructose corn syrup	A highly concentrated syrup of mostly fructose and some glucose; very prevalent in soft drinks and other processed foods.
White grape juice	A highly purified fructose solution; virtually no other nutrients are present.
Mannitol, Sorbitol, Xylitol	Sugar alcohols derived from fruit or produced from dextrose. All three contain the same number of calories as sugar (4 calories per gram). Sugar alcohols are more slowly absorbed than sugar is. For this reason, the sugar alcohols are thought to be better than sugar for diabetics. Sugar alcohols do not promote tooth decay, unlike sugar.

WHEN GOOD CARBS GO BAD

Recognize that any good carb can be degraded into a bad carb through processing; through the addition of sugar, fat, or additives; or through overcooking. A good example is the potato. What starts out as a highly nutritious, filling nutrient-rich carb when baked, morphs quickly into a miserable, greasy, high-calorie, bad carb when made into french fries or potato chips. The point is, eating mostly good carbs—foods that are natural and wholesome—will help keep you in peak health.

SUMMING UP

*Carbohydrates can be evaluated in at least three differ*ent ways, all useful in their various applications. As you study the three scorecards, you can see that good carbs share certain characteristics, regardless of the scorecard applied. Good carbs are:

- Plentiful in vitamins, minerals, antioxidants, and phytochemicals.

- High in disease-preventing fiber.

- Free of added sugar and harmful additives.

- Pure, unrefined, and minimally processed.

- Generally helpful in controlling blood sugar and insulin levels.

- Protective against an array of diseases.

As you make your daily food choices, keep these characteristics in mind. Your body prefers good carbs and uses them so much more efficiently than it uses processed, chemical-laden bad carbs, such as refined cereals, commercially baked goods, or fat, sugar, and additive-loaded packaged foods. Bad carbs are nutritionally bankrupt and associated with various health problems. Good carbs are bursting with nutrients, each put to use in building and healing the body.

THREE

Healthy Bites:
The Twenty-five Super Carbs

*Without question, carbohydrates are a vital food for sup-*plying energy and supporting good health. And as you have seen, some carbs are more desirable than others. But even among those good carbs, some deserve to go to the head of the line, because they are brimming with natural chemicals and other nutrients that are exceptionally strong guardians of health.

Here are twenty-five super carbs to stock in your kitchen in order to boost your immune system, protect yourself against disease, and perform at your very best. Each is a winner on all three carb scorecards discussed in the previous chapter. Make it a habit to serve up a variety of these foods, along with other good carbs, every day of the week.

1. Apple

There's a reason why the old saying "an apple a day keeps the doctor away" has had such a long life: Apples have a

slew of health benefits all attributable to their high phytochemical and high fiber contents.

One of the major phytochemicals in apples is quercetin.
Research indicates that quercetin deters the changes that
make prostate cells cancerous and might retard the cancer's spread. It also might reduce the risk of lung cancer.
A 25-year follow-up study involving nearly 10,000 Finn-
ish men showed a reduced risk for lung cancer in cases
where the consumption of apples was high. In animals,
quercetin has also been found to inhibit the growth of
melanoma, a deadly form of skin cancer.

Apples are high in fiber, too, with one fruit supplying
5 grams of fiber. Roughly 80 percent of that fiber is soluble and, thus, heart-protective; the rest is insoluble, the
form believed to exert an anticancer benefit. You'll also
find plenty of vitamin A, B vitamins, and various minerals
in apples.

An apple a day keeps the dentist away, too. When you
crunch down on an apple, it scours away some of the
bacteria and plaque that adheres to your teeth.

2. Artichokes

How fondly I remember my favorite lunch as a child—
boiled artichokes, their tender leaves dipped in my
mother's homemade mayonnaise. I'd pull the leaves between my teeth (there's an "art" to eating artichokes) and
feast on their delicious pulp.

Little did I know then that I was dining not only on a
delectable vegetable but also on one whose leaves are
chock-full of phytochemicals. Among the phytochemicals
in artichoke leaves are flavonoids, plant pigments that act
as antioxidants; fructo-ogliosaccharides (FOS), a group of
beneficial nondigestible carbohydrates; caffeoylquinic acids, which save cells from free radical damage; and luteo-

lin, an antioxidant that appears to reduce levels of LDL (bad) cholesterol.

Artichoke (*Cynara scolymus*) is a member of the aster family, to which daisies, dandelions, chrysanthemums, and the milk thistle plant also belong. What you see in the supermarket is actually the flower of this plant.

Since ancient times, artichoke leaf has been used medicinally as a "choleretic" (bile increasing) and as a diuretic. In folk medicine, it is a well-known cure for digestive problems. Over the past few decades, mounting scientific evidence has verified the validity of these traditional claims, plus it has shown the artichoke leaf to be a bonafide treatment for other conditions, namely high cholesterol and liver problems.

If you've never prepared an artichoke, it's very easy to do. Simply boil the artichokes in a large saucepan of water (add 2 tablespoons vinegar for flavoring) for about 45 minutes. Dip the leaves in your favorite low-fat or reduced-fat salad dressing, and enjoy. Canned artichoke hearts make great additions to salads.

3. Avocado

Okay, I know you're thinking that an avocado is a fat and, yes, it is extremely high in *healthy* fats. But the avocado, technically a fruit, is a mixture of protein, fat— and carbohydrate—so it's difficult to pigeonhole it into any one nutrient category. There are two varieties of avocado—Florida and California—and both are equally loaded with nutrients.

Avocados are also a valuable source of fiber. The California avocado yields 8 grams of fiber; the Florida variety, 16 grams. Their antioxidant content is second to none. Avocados contain glutathione (more than three times that found in other fruits), and are the highest fruit source of lutein. Glutathione detoxifies cancer-causing agents. Lu-

tein is best known for preventing eye diseases, and it
might guard against cancers of the colon, lung, and breast.
Avocados also contain more vitamin E than any other
fruit.

People used to shun the avocado because of its fat, but
now we know better. The fat in this fruit is of two major
types: monounsaturated, which is known to keep cholesterol levels in check, and beta-sitosterol, also a good cholesterol regulator.

4. Beets

If you're like most people, beets probably aren't a mealtime staple at your house, although they should be. This
root vegetable is a nutritional treasure trove. A cup of
cooked sliced beets, for example, yields 3 grams of fiber.
Plus, beets are loaded with disease-fighting antioxidants.
Also going for beets: One serving of beets provides more
than a third of your daily requirement for folate. You
probably know this nutrient best as folic acid, but folate
is the form found in food; folic acid is the supplement
form. Folate, a member of the family of B vitamins, is
critical for the synthesis, repair, and functioning of DNA,
the genetic material of cells. Folate is a super-critical nutrient that might reduce your risk of heart disease, stroke,
and colon cancer.

5. Berries

Blueberries, strawberries, raspberries, and blackberries are
among the healthiest fruit carbohydrates you can eat because they're loaded with antioxidants that protect you
from heart disease, cancer, and many other diseases. One
of the most protective substances in berries is a phytochemical called ellagic acid, which prevents toxic chemicals from damaging cells. Not only that, it helps initiate

a process that causes cancer cells to commit suicide.

Blueberries, in particular, have been identified as a fruit that enhances age-related short-term memory, says a Tufts University study conducted with rats. Much like people, rats become more forgetful as they get older, unable to find their way through mazes they once knew how to navigate. But when they were fed extracts of blueberries for two months, they actually improved their ability to navigate through mazes! Not only that, the rats' balance, coordination, and running speed improved. In similar tests, strawberries worked, too, but not as well. Scientists speculate that antioxidants in blueberries reduce inflammation, a process that might harm brain tissue as we get older.

6. Broccoli Sprouts

Although broccoli is certainly a highly nutritious carbohydrate, its forerunner, broccoli sprouts, are even more healthful. Several years ago, scientists at Johns Hopkins University in Baltimore discovered that, cup for cup, broccoli sprouts have 10 to 100 times more anticancer substances in them than regular broccoli. These substances are phytochemicals called isothiocyanates. They work by activating the antioxidant glutathione, which detoxifies carcinogens.

Both broccoli and broccoli sprouts contain a phytochemical called sulforaphane, which also protects cells against cancer. Sulforaphane has another bonus: It appears to eradicate a bacteria in the stomach called *H. pylori*, which causes ulcers.

If you want to start reaping the benefits these sprouts offer, eat about a cup and half a day. That's the recommended amount for good health. Don't forget to eat your broccoli, too. With its fiber, B vitamins, beta-carotene, and vitamin C (one of the most important antioxidants and cancer fighters), it's worth piling on your plate.

7. Brown Rice

When you want some rice, one of your best choices is brown rice. Compared to white rice, which has been stripped of nutrients, brown rice has its bran layer still intact and is, thus, a top source of B vitamins, including thiamin (vitamin B_1); the minerals calcium, phosphorus, and iron; and fiber. Brown rice is also a good source of vitamin E.

8. Bulgur Wheat

Less familiar among most good carbs, bulgur wheat is a form of whole wheat that can be eaten as a breakfast food or as a delicious side dish at lunch or dinner. You can cook bulgur wheat as you do rice or simply soak it in water or broth. Bulgur is often used as a meat extender or meat substitute in vegetarian cooking. It is best known as the chief ingredient in tabouli salad, a popular Mideastern dish. Nutritionally, bulgur wheat is high in insoluble fiber (5 grams per serving) and is loaded with B vitamins, phosphorus, zinc, copper, iron, and magnesium.

9. Cabbage

The world's oldest cultivated vegetable, cabbage has today become known as an anticancer vegetable. It is high in the cancer-fighting phytochemical glutathione, as well as vitamin A, calcium, and fiber—all nutrients that appear to have cancer-protective effects, particularly in lowering the risk of stomach, breast, and intestinal cancers.

10. Concord Grape Juice

This form of grape juice has more antioxidants than any other juice. In studies, it helps thwart the oxidation of artery-damaging LDL cholesterol—a process caused by free radicals. When LDL cholesterol is oxidized by free radicals, white blood cells in artery linings start attracting excessive amounts of LDL. The oxidized LDL forms fatty streaks on the inner arterial walls, and these streaks become the foundation of atherosclerosis, the abnormal thickening of the arteries that leads to heart disease. There are many different kinds of grape juice on supermarket shelves, and few offer the natural health protection of Concord grape juice. Be sure to look for a brand that specifies that it is 100 percent Concord grape juice.

11. Garlic

In ancient times, garlic was believed to scare off vampires, but now we know that it wards off a great deal more. This centuries-old remedy might have preventive and curative properties in a wide range of ailments, including heart disease, cancer, and immune system disorders. Garlic, it seems, contains more than 200 biologically active compounds that appear to positively alter the course of many illnesses. It is also an antibacterial and an antifungal agent. The best way to secure garlic's healing power is to mash it or mince it prior to adding it to recipes.

12. Greens

There is a long list of green leafy vegetables that are phenomenal in the health benefits they confer. Beet greens, collard greens, dandelion greens, kale, spinach, and turnip greens are just a few of the names on this all-star list of nutritional heroes. What they have in common is their wealth of beta-carotene, vitamin C, folate, iron, and other minerals. These foods also contain phytochemicals that help protect your eyes. Make it a point to eat more green leafy vegetables every day—in salads, soups, or stews.

13. Kiwifruit

Used to be, kiwifruit was relegated to garnish status for fruit trays, but not anymore. Kiwifruit has been promoted to the position of super fruit—and for good reason. This fuzzy little green fruit is packed with vitamin C (more than double what you find in an orange). In fact, one medium kiwifruit provides 120 milligrams of vitamin C; that's twice the daily requirement. For weight control, few fruits beat the kiwifruit. One fruit has just 46 calories.

14. Legumes

Technically an edible seed with a pod, legumes represent a huge family of nutritious vegetables, including beans, peas, and lentils. These vegetables are near-perfect foods, too, containing not only a lot of complex carbohydrates, but plenty of protein as well. As such, they can be used as a meat substitute in vegetarian diets.

Legumes are among the carbs highest in fiber, with 7 grams on average per cup. The soluble fiber contained in legumes helps lower cholesterol. A tip: Don't toss out the liquid in canned beans. Use it for soups, because there is soluble fiber dissolved in this liquid. Legumes are also loaded with iron and the B vitamins folate, thiamin, riboflavin, and niacin.

15. Oatmeal

Oatmeal might not be the most exciting breakfast cereal to wake up to, but it certainly is one of the most healthy. Oatmeal contains a soluble fiber called beta-glucan, which, like a nutritional housecleaner, sweeps out cholesterol-forming particles from your body before they can turn into full-blown artery-clogging cholesterol. Eating oatmeal on a regular basis has been proven to naturally lower dangerous cholesterol and reduce blood pressure. Oatmeal is also one of the few foods that is naturally rich in vitamin E.

Not all oatmeal is alike when it comes to nutritional value, however. Rolled oats, old-fashioned oats, and steel-cut oats are nutritionally superior to the quick or instant varieties.

16. Onions

Yes, onions stink up your breath, but from a health perspective, the stench is worth it. This sometimes unpopular vegetable is beneficial for heart health. It prevents arteries from clogging and contains beneficial substances that stop the formation of dangerous blood clots, which can lead to heart attacks.

Onions contain phytochemicals called saponins, which prevent cancer cells from multiplying, and allylic sulfides, which usher carcinogens from your body, decrease tumor reproduction, and fortify your immune system. Onions are also high in quercetin, an anticancer phytochemical.

17. Oranges

Oranges and other citrus fruits are a storehouse of nutrients, from phytochemicals to vitamins. Best known for their vitamin C content, these fruits also contain phenolics, which are phytochemicals that neutralize carcinogens and stimulate the production of cancer-fighting glutathione. Oranges are a known source of limonene, a phytochemical that stops damaged cells from the uncontrolled growth that can lead to cancer. Another protective nutrient found in oranges is folate, a B vitamin.

Citrus fruits are high in substances called flavonoids, found abundantly in vegetables, grains, tea, and wine. More than 5,000 flavonoids have been discovered in na-

ture, and many are responsible for the bright colors of the
fruits and vegetables you eat. Flavonoids are also essential
for the proper absorption of vitamin C. In fact, flavonoids
are what make natural vitamin C (found in foods) more
effective than synthetic supplemental vitamin C by improving and prolonging the function of the vitamin.

18. Pineapple

Probably the world's most favorite tropical fruit, pineap-
ples pack a huge nutritional wallop. They're high in vitamin C, fiber, and the mineral manganese, which protects
both your bones and your heart. This delicious fruit is
chock-full of a natural enzyme called bromelain, a known
anti-inflammatory and a "mucolytic," which means it
eliminates the abnormal accumulation of mucus in tissues.
Indeed, bromelain has wide-ranging health benefits: It appears to alleviate diarrhea by healing the mucosa of the
colon, help prevent heart disease by interfering with the
formation of abnormal clots, and possibly stave off cancer
due to an antitumor effect. To capitalize on the benefits
of pineapple, it's best to eat it fresh, because the processing required to can the fruit destroys most of its bromelain.

19. Red Pepper

When scientists at Cornell University analyzed the antioxidant activity of ten common vegetables in their lab a
few years ago, they discovered that red peppers had the
highest activity, followed by broccoli, carrots, spinach,
cabbage, yellow onions, celery, potatoes, lettuce, and cucumbers. In addition, red peppers were among the top
three vegetables found to interfere with the proliferation
of human liver cancer cells that had been isolated in a lab
dish. Spinach performed the best, followed by cabbage,

with red peppers in third place. What this study hints at
is that red peppers are a vegetable with much curative and
preventive powers.

20. Romaine Lettuce

When you select a lettuce with dark green leaves, such as
romaine lettuce, you're getting a real nutritional bargain.
Romaine lettuce, the mainstay of Caesar salads, is an excellent source of vitamin C, vitamin A, and folate. Further, it has eight times more beta-carotene and twice as
much calcium as iceberg lettuce.

21. Sweet Potato

If you had to eat just one vegetable, it might be a good
idea to choose the sweet potato. Ounce for ounce, it is
one of the most nutritious vegetables around and loaded
with beta-carotene, which converts to vitamin A in your
body. Vitamin A is an important antioxidant that strength-
ens your immune system against bacterial and viral diseases as well as cancer. Sweet potatoes also supply
cholesterol-lowering fiber, vitamin C, vitamin E, and the
B vitamin thiamin. Although sweet, these spuds are not
at all high in calories, providing roughly 120 per medium-
size potato.

22. Tomato

Pass the ketchup, the spaghetti sauce, and the tomatoes—
please! Tomatoes and tomato products are the primary
sources of lycopene, a powerful carotenoid that works
forcefully as an antioxidant fighting off disease-causing
free radicals. Lycopene appears to be highly protective
against cancers of the colon, bladder, and pancreas, but it
is particularly noteworthy for its role in preventing pros-

tate cancer. In a diet study sponsored by the National Cancer Institute, researchers identified lycopene as being extremely powerful against prostate cancer. Those individuals who consumed greater than ten servings of tomato-based foods per week had a significantly decreased risk of developing prostate cancer when compared to those who ate fewer than 1½ servings per week. Tomatoes are also a rich source of vitamin C and many other phytochemicals.

23. Wheat Bran·

Sprinkling a few tablespoons of raw wheat bran on your cereal in the morning does a world of good for your digestive system. Wheat bran acts as a natural laxative, promoting regularity. For women, there's an added plus of eating wheat bran: It helps move excess estrogen from the body. That's important, because too much estrogen in the body is a risk factor for breast cancer.

24. Winter Squash

Acorn, butternut, hubbard, and banana squash are all well-known members of the winter squash family. Like most orange-, yellow-, and red-colored vegetables, winter squash is high in key carotenoids, including alpha-carotene, beta-carotene, lutein, and zeaxanthin.

Alpha-carotene shows promise in stalling the growth of certain malignant tumors and might be protective against breast cancer. Butternut and hubbard squashes are good sources of alpha-carotene. Beta-carotene reduces the risk of cancers of the colon, rectum, breast, uterus, prostate, and lung. All varieties of winter squash contain significant amounts of beta-carotene.

Lutein, better known for preventing eye diseases, might guard against cancer of the colon, lung, and breast. Its

less-well-known companion carotenoid, zeaxanthin, is
linked to a lower risk of breast, cervical, and colon cancers. Both carotenoids are being investigated for their role
in preventing skin cancer. Acorn squash, which is also
very high in fiber, contains lutein and zeaxanthin.

25. Yogurt

Yogurt is produced by fermenting milk with a mixture of
bacteria and yeasts. The process yields not only a delicious, custardlike treat, but also a food that is brimming
with "probiotics" (a term that means "favoring life"). Probiotics are healthy bacteria that help maintain the health
of the digestive tract, preventing the growth of yeast, sal-
monella, *E. coli*, and other nasty germs. Among the most
well-known probiotic is *L. acidophilus*, which is plentiful
in yogurt. In numerous studies, it has demonstrated antitumor activity, particularly against colon cancer. And, in
at least one study, it prevented recurring tumors in bladder-
cancer patients.

The healthy bacteria in yogurt also have an immune-
boosting effect. In a study conducted at the University of
California–Davis, researchers found that people who ate
2 cups of yogurt a day had fewer colds.

Yogurt is also rich in bone-building calcium, B vitamins, vitamins A and D, and protein. It is helpful in treating high cholesterol, digestive disorders, and kidney
problems.

Footnote: Be sure to avoid yogurts sweetened with
added sugar. The best option is to buy plain yogurt and
sweeten it yourself with low-sugar or nonsugar jam.

Variety Is the Spice of Life

Along with an active lifestyle, one of the ways to get a
superfit body is by eating a diet that includes these super

carbs as well as other good carbs. Doing so ensures that you get the greatest variety possible of health-building nutrients. Just remember: Every time you pile these good carbs on your plate, you're serving up a lot more than meets the eye.

PART II

Your Good Carb Prescription for Health

FOUR

Your Brain on Carbs

We don't often think of food as a drug, but food does indeed have druglike effects on the body. It is within the brain that food, particularly carbohydrates, is used to manufacture important brain chemicals called neurotransmitters that, in their ebb and flow, govern your mind, your memory, and even your very behavior in ways that might be quite dramatic. This whole notion that carbohydrates can affect your brain and behavior as powerfully as a drug came to national prominence in the late 1970s, when San Francisco supervisor Dan White claimed that a junk-food diet of Twinkies and Coca Cola put him into a heightened emotional state and deepened his depression when he shot and killed the mayor and another city employee. The defense worked. The jury found White guilty, but of the lesser charge of manslaughter and sentenced him to six years in prison. The celebrated case has since come to be known as the "Twinkie Defense."

To a great degree, the foundations of good, stable mental fitness rest on what you eat. A healthful diet, devoid of highly processed foods, supplies your brain with the nutrients and energy it needs for optimal functioning and psychological health. And certainly, eating too many high-sugar junk foods on a regular basis can be mentally detrimental. Sugar drives your blood sugar up quite rapidly, but this reaction is followed by a fast crash downward as your blood sugar plummets. Low blood sugar, or hypoglycemia, has a depressant effect on the body; it makes you feel blue and out of sorts. However, the association between criminal behavior and the consumption of refined sugar (the Twinkie Defense) has never been verified.

In the information that follows, you'll learn why eating certain carbs (even a little bit of sugar), in the right amounts, holds some of the most powerful secrets to exceptional mental fitness.

CARBOHYDRATES: THE BRAIN FUEL

From the cereal you eat for breakfast to the baked potato you have for dinner, carbs are the leading nutrient fuel for your brain. Your brain uses glucose from the breakdown of carbohydrates almost exclusively in regulating everything mental, from learning to memory to mood. Without ongoing replenishment of glucose, your brain would be deprived of glucose in a mere ten minutes, and your mental power would suffer greatly.

As glucose circulates in your bloodstream, ready to be taken up by cells for energy, your brain gets first dibs on it before any other organ does. And if for some reason glucose is in short supply, your brain will commandeer processes that convert other nutrients into glucose. The health and performance of your brain depend on a readily available supply of glucose, and you can boost your brainpower enormously by adequately fueling yourself with carbs. Carbs play a central role in alertness, concentration, mood, and memory, as well as in protection against a number of brain-damaging diseases. (Some of the important effects of carbohydrates on your brain are listed in the following box.)

EFFECTS OF CARBOHYDRATES ON YOUR BRAIN

- Fuels the brain for mental activity
- Increases the production of important brain chemicals such as serotonin
- Produces feelings of calmness
- Reduces anxiety
- Induces sleep
- Heightens recall
- Suppresses the appetite

MIND POWER AND MENTAL CONCENTRATION

Maybe you might have to be on your mental toes for an important meeting. Maybe you are scheduled to take an exam. Maybe you are set to learn a new task on your job. Or maybe you're driving long hours toward a destination. Whatever the situation, you need needle-sharp focus and quick response time. You'll be gratified to know that carbohydrates are your knight in shining armor in this regard.

Carbohydrates are powerful nutrients for boosting alertness and concentration, as long as you select the right ones and in the right amounts. When you are learning a new task, your brain begins to rapidly take up glucose from circulation. Scientists believe that, during a learning activity, glucose may activate the release of a neurotransmitter called acetylcholine to help retain memory. Manufactured from the B vitamin choline, this neurotransmitter is involved mostly in learning and memory. So if you must stay alert through the day, make sure you're fueling your brain with at least one or two servings of good carbs at each meal.

If some of these carbs are rich in vitamin C, you'll boost your alertness even more. Vitamin C increases levels of the neurotransmitter norepinedrine in your brain. Norepinedrine helps you stay alert and motivated. Good choices include citrus fruits, strawberries, kiwifruit, and sweet peppers.

If your powers of concentration need rejuvenating, here's a menu filled with alertness-boosting foods, including carbs, along with information on why they work. (Foods marked by an asterisk indicate that the food is a carbohydrate.)

The Alertness Diet

Breakfast

    2 scrambled eggs

    *1 slice whole-wheat bread with 1 pat butter or margarine

    *1 cup Concord grape juice

    1 cup coffee

Mid-Morning Snack

    *1 medium apple

Lunch

4 ounces tuna salad (2 to 3 cups mixed *salad vegetables, including 1 *tomato, cut into wedges)

2 tablespoons reduced-fat French dressing

1 cup coffee

Mid-Afternoon Snack

*1 medium orange

2 tablespoons peanuts

Dinner

4 to 5 ounces grilled lean beef

*1 cup cooked mixed vegetables

*½ acorn squash

*1 cup skim milk

Why It Works

- The apple, peanuts, and tomato are loaded with boron.
  Research indicates that people given additional boron
  score higher on tests that measure attention and memory.

- The whole-wheat toast is an excellent source of glucose.

- The orange is high in vitamin C, which helps synthesize norepinedrine.

- The lunch in this menu is low in carbohydrates. Here's
  the reason why: Too many carbs at lunch impairs at-

tention span and reaction time. To increase alertness, stick to high-protein lunches. Have coffee with lunch if you want to get rid of post-lunch mental slumps. Coffee is a source of caffeine, which boosts alertness.

- The large salad at lunch contains potassium. If you don't get enough of this mineral in your diet, you could have trouble concentrating.

- The grape juice, acorn squash, and other vegetables are chock-full of brain-protecting antioxidants. Concord grape juice, in particular, is one of the most antioxidant-rich foods you can eat.

- The grilled lean beef supplies iron, a mineral important to brain function because it boosts concentration and enhances learning.

CARBOHYDRATE MOOD BOOSTERS

Many experts believe that you can defeat a bad mood with what you eat, as long as you select the right foods—those that have a positive effect on brain chemistry. Carbohydrates just happen to be a key "nutrient tranquilizer." If you'd love to soothe jangled nerves, chase away the blues, or lift your spirits, look to carbs for a mood-boosting remedy. A diet rich in carbohydrates can help you feel relaxed and less stressed out, because carbohydrates are indirectly involved with elevating a neurotransmitter called serotonin. Serotonin is known as the "happiness neurotransmitter" because it is associated with tranquility, calm, and emotional well-being.

Eating carbohydrates kicks off a cascade of events that produce serotonin. This process starts when you have a meal that contains protein. Protein foods such as milk and poultry are rich sources of the amino acid tryptophan, a building block of serotonin.

Protein foods contain other amino acids besides tryptophan and in larger amounts. To reach the brain, these amino acids must cross the "blood-brain barrier," a protective network of tightly knit cells lining the blood vessels of the brain. These cells are trusty, vigilant receptionists that screen substances for entry into the brain and bar the door to unwelcome toxins. Those substances that do get in are ferried across the blood-brain barrier by special carrier molecules. Like a passenger vying for a seat on a crowded bus, tryptophan has to compete with five larger amino acids for a ride over. Consequently, not much tryptophan enters, so very little serotonin is synthesized in the brain in response to a high-protein meal.

However, if carbohydrate foods are eaten with protein foods, the carbohydrate helps deliver more tryptophan to the brain. Carbohydrate triggers the release of insulin, which drives amino acids right into brain cells. Thus, eating high-carbohydrate meals—rather than high-protein meals—ships tryptophan into the brain, where it can be eventually converted into serotonin to boost your mood.

To sum up, the process works like this: A high-carbohydrate meal triggers the release of insulin, and more tryptophan can then enter the brain. Tryptophan is used to make serotonin, and the result of more serotonin is a feeling of calmness.

Incidentally, if you crave carbohydrates, it could be because your brain is crying out for more serotonin. (For an explanation of why you crave carbs, see the following box.)

Do You Crave Carbohydrates?

You know the feeling, that I just gotta have a doughnut . . . a chocolate candy bar . . . some Ben & Jerry's ice cream. Technically, this overpowering desire is called "carbohydrate craving," and it has a biochemical basis. Usually, we start craving carbs because our brain is putting in an order for more serotonin precursors, or building blocks. The chief building block for serotonin is the amino acid tryptophan, available from protein but shuttled into the brain by insulin, which is triggered by eating carbohydrates. So the cravings are essentially a shout for more tryptophan.

Some people are more likely than others to get carbohydrate cravings. They include:

• Those who are overweight or obese. People who are obese often suffer from "insulin resistance," the inability of the body's cells to properly use insulin to drive various substances into cells, including tryptophan. Consequently, not much tryptophan gets shipped into the brain to make serotonin. Trimming down to a smaller size through exercise and diet will resolve insulin resistance and, with it, carbohydrate cravings.

• Women with premenstrual syndrome (PMS). A woman's craving for sweets can intensify during the premenstrual phase of her monthly cycle—a reaction that might also be attributed to fluctuating levels of serotonin in the brain. A highly craved food during this time is chocolate—and yes, it works to ease the depression and anxiety associated with PMS. Chocolate helps synthesize serotonin, possibly because it is high in sugar or some other unknown chemical. Rather than munch on chocolate or other sweets, it's preferable to reach for good carbs such as whole-wheat bread, pasta, or cereals to soothe the premenstrual blues. One study found that eating a carbohydrate-rich, low-protein dinner improved depression, tension, anger, sadness, fatigue, and alertness among a group of women suffering from PMS.

• People with seasonal affective disorder (SAD), a form of depression that strikes 10 to 25 million Americans, usually in the fall and winter. This extreme form of the wintertime blues is thought to stem from abnormalities in the brain chemicals. Low levels of light

in the winter disturb the balance of brain chemicals being released, particularly serotonin. Treatments for SAD generally include bright light therapy, exercise, and antidepressant therapy to
restore normal levels of serotonin in the brain. Appropriate treatment helps alleviate the cravings.

One of the best mood-boosting carbs you can eat is
whole-grain bread. Its attraction lies in its mixture of carbohydrates and amino acids, a combo that allows the most
efficient delivery of tryptophan to the brain. In fact,
whole-grain bread is a near-perfect blend of proteins and
carbohydrates that practically ensures that your brain will
get enough tryptophan to manufacture serotonin.

Another great mood-boosting carb is the banana. Bananas are well endowed with magnesium, a mineral de-
pleted by stress. When you're chronically stressed out,
your body starts churning out more stress hormones, high
levels of which cause magnesium to be flushed from cells.
This can lead to all kinds of problems, including vulner-
ability to viruses and mood-sapping fatigue. Bananas are
also loaded with tryptophan, the amino acid that improves
serotonin metabolism.

Although generally dubbed a "bad carb," particularly
in excess amounts, pure sugar is a natural upper in one
important regard. Its sweet taste—the sensation you feel
when you eat it—triggers the release of feel-good chemicals in your body called endorphins. Researchers have
actually observed that the moods of depressed patients
brightened considerably when they were fed high-sugar
meals. Think twice, however, before popping sugar cubes
for a high. A sugar overload will lead to weight gain, and
putting on weight is a depressing predicament for plenty
of people. Plus, it can lead to mood-deflating hypoglycemia (low blood sugar).

Many of the good carbs listed in this book are packed

with B vitamins, which play a critical role in brain function, from manufacturing neurotransmitters to releasing energy in your brain cells. Two B vitamins of note are folate and thiamin. Found in orange juice, green leafy vegetables, and fortified bread and breakfast cereals, folate has been shown in research to be effective for easing depression. To get the mood-boosting benefits of folate, try to eat a cup of spinach or other green leafy vegetable, several times a week.

Nicknamed the "morale vitamin" because of its beneficial effect on mental attitude, thiamin is plentiful in good carbs such as wheat germ, bran, brown rice, and whole grains. Not only does this important B vitamin help alleviate depression, it can also improve your capacity to learn and grasp new information.

Besides the mood-lifting carbs already discussed, others include corn, dry cereals, green leafy vegetables, muffins, oatmeal, pasta, potatoes, and rice. Here's a sample menu that might help overturn a down-in-the-dumps mood. It is high in good-mood carbs. (Foods marked by an asterisk indicate that the food is a carbohydrate.)

The Blues-Banishing Diet

Breakfast

 *1 slice whole-wheat toast

 ½ cup cooked *oatmeal, sprinkled with 1 tablespoon *bran and 1 tablespoon *wheat germ

 *½ cup skim milk

 *½ grapefruit

Mid-Morning Snack

 *1 cup fruit-flavored yogurt

Lunch

*Vegetable pasta: 1¼ cup pasta topped with 1 cup assorted vegetables and ¾ cup marinara sauce

1 small serving *spinach salad with 1 tablespoon ranch dressing

Mid-Afternoon Snack

*1 granola bar

*1 banana

Dinner

4 to 5 ounces grilled salmon

*½ cup brown rice, with *½ cup red beans

*½ avocado with 1 tablespoon Italian dressing

Bedtime Snack

*½ cup frozen yogurt or sherbet

Why It Works

• The breakfast featured here is high in carbohydrate, which increases brain levels of serotonin, the neurotransmitter responsible for elevating your mood.

• The salmon is loaded with mood-stabilizing omega-3 fatty acids, which play a role in mental well-being by raising levels of serotonin in the brain.

• The pasta suggested for lunch will help prevent serotonin levels from dipping too low.

• The tomato-based marinara sauce is rich in selenium, a mineral needed in the diet to prevent depression. Other depression-defeating nutrients include vitamin C in the grapefruit, folate in the spinach and avocado, vitamin B_{12} in the fish and dairy products, niacin in vegetables and dairy products, and calcium and vitamin D in the dairy products. Brown rice is high in thiamin, a B vitamin that helps reduce mood-sapping fatigue.

• The protein-rich foods in this menu—fish, dairy products, brown rice, and red beans—supply various types of good-mood amino acids. The fish, beans, and oats (in the oatmeal and granola bar), for example, are high in tryptophan, a building block of serotonin. These same foods are also rich in tyrosine and phenylalanine, two amino acids that ward off bad moods.

• The frozen yogurt or sherbet in the bedtime snack is high in glucose and protein, which will enhance the production of mood-lifting serotonin.

MEMORY: WHEN A SIMPLE SUGAR (GLUCOSE) TURNS GOOD

*Feeling like the absentminded professor lately? Fortu*nately, you can bring back a faltering memory by populating your diet with memory-boosting foods, and one of the most surprising is the simple sugar, glucose. Through studies with animals and humans, scientists have discovered that a jolt of glucose, taken after fasting or following a meal, will improve long-term memory, the part of your memory that stores most of everything you know.

Case in point: In a University of Virginia study, investigators served a group of college students lemonade containing 50 grams of glucose (about 200 calories' worth of sugar), then gave them a number of cognitive tests. Drinking the glucose-spiked lemonade greatly enhanced the students' mental performance, particularly on a reading retention exercise. Other fascinating research has found that people with Alzheimer's disease, Down's syndrome, and head injuries perform much better on mental tests when given glucose. Scientists do not know exactly why or how glucose enhances memory so well, but investigations into this benefit are ongoing. One good source of liquid glucose is a sports drink such as Gatorade. Used to replace lost fluid after intense exercise or strenuous work, sports drinks are a mixture of water, carbohydrate (mostly glucose), and minerals called electrolytes.

Glucose as a memory enhancer certainly looks promising, and if used for this purpose, it could be classified as a "good carb." But before you rush out and get some sugary lemonade or glucose-containing sports drinks, let me caution you that to date no one knows what the optimum dose is for mental performance. You might be able to chug 50 grams of glucose in a beverage with no problems at all, but someone else might get high blood sugar due to metabolic differences. So do some experimenting to see how much is right for you.

Here's a typical menu to un-muddle your mind and enhance your memory. (Foods marked by an asterisk indicate that the food is a carbohydrate.)

The Remembrance Menu

Breakfast

*½ cup cream of wheat, sprinkled with 2 tablespoons *wheat bran

2 eggs, any style

*½ cup blueberries

1 cup green tea, iced or hot

Mid-Morning Snack

*8 ounces tomato juice blended with 1 tablespoon brewer's yeast

3 tablespoons almonds or walnuts

Lunch

Tuna salad on a bed of *green leafy lettuce

1 banana

1 cup green tea, iced or hot

Mid-Afternoon Snack

*4 whole-wheat crackers

2 ounces sliced turkey

*1 cup glucose-containing sports drink

Dinner

12 baked oysters

*½ cup brown rice

*1 cup cauliflower

1 cup fruit-flavored yogurt

Why It Works

• Eggs and dairy products are excellent sources of choline for producing acetylcholine, the memory neurotransmitter.

• In recent animal studies, blueberries have been identified as a fruit that enhances short-term memory. The fruit is well endowed with antioxidants and phyto-chemicals (plant chemicals) that protect the brain against degeneration. Scientists speculate that antioxidants in blueberries reduce inflammation, a process that might harm brain tissue as we get older. Blueberries are among the richest fruit sources of antioxidants. Tomato juice and green leafy vegetables also contain important antioxidants.

- Folate is present in brewer's yeast and green leafy lettuce. Among its many other duties in brain health, folate helps prevent dementia.

- Brewer's yeast and brown rice are a top sources of thiamin (vitamin B_1), which is required for the synthesis of acetylcholine and is involved in improving learning capacity.

- Tuna, turkey, whole wheat, eggs, brewer's yeast, bananas, and cauliflower all contain vitamin B_6, which helps boost long-term memory.

- Tuna is high in docosahexaenoic acid, or DHA, a key memory-enhancing fat. Because of its importance in human brain tissue, DHA might help prevent degenerative brain diseases such as dementia, memory loss, and Alzheimer's disease.

- Oysters, tuna, and wheat bran are loaded with zinc, a mineral that plays a vital role in memory formation and retention.

- The fish, poultry, and brewer's yeast in this menu provide the B vitamin niacin, which dilates blood vessels so more blood, oxygen, and nutrients can reach and nourish your brain.

- Nuts such as almonds or walnuts are good sources of

vitamin E, which appears to protect against degenerative brain diseases such as Alzheimer's disease.

• Drinking green tea is recommended for memory preservation. It protects against cognitive decline in the elderly by reducing bodily levels of cholesterol and homocysteine, a harmful protein that has been implicated in heart disease. Both substances are associated with elevated amounts of beta amyloid peptides, proteins that form plaques in the brain and lead to Alzheimer's disease (see below).

BRAIN PROTECTION WITH GOOD CARBS

Unfortunately, your brain is vulnerable to various illnesses, some of them serious, debilitating, and life-threatening. One of the scariest is dementia. Dementia is a condition in which you gradually lose the ability to remember, think, reason, interact socially, and care for yourself. It is not a disease, but rather a cluster of symptoms triggered by diseases or conditions that adversely affect the brain. Some of these triggers can be treated and are referred to as "reversible" dementia; others cannot be cured and are termed "irreversible" dementia. Examples of irreversible dementia include Alzheimer's disease and multi-infarct dementia.

Reversible Dementia

Two forms of reversible dementia are nutrition related. "Nutritional" dementia is one of these. Virtually any shortfall of nutrients, particularly the B vitamins, will cause dementia. Among other duties, B vitamins are an important factor in regulating the health of your nerves, so it should come as no surprise that they are intimately involved in the workings of the brain. B vitamins are most plentiful in whole grains, a group of good carbs. But if your diet is too high in refined foods with lots of added sugar, you could be putting yourself at risk of a B vitamin deficiency, because sugar destroys these important brain-protective nutrients.

Another form of reversible dementia has to do with alcohol dependence. Alcohol, a bad carb, is essentially a toxin that, if abused, can damage your brain, cause memory loss, and induce dementia. In fact, chronic alcoholism can cause a type of amnesia in which the brain is unable to form new memories. Treatment for alcohol dependence and the dementia it causes is very straightforward: abstinence.

Alzheimer's Disease

Among the most feared of all brain diseases is Alzheimer's disease. If it strikes, you gradually lose your mind, your memory, and the ability to recognize your loved ones. In the advanced stages of the disease, you become totally dependent on others for your care. Alzheimer's disease is unusual in that it can be definitively diagnosed only after death through an autopsy of the brain, although mental functioning tests can be administered to detect the possibility of the disease.

Happily though, huge strides have been made in learning how to delay and even prevent the symptoms of this horrifying disease, as well as how to treat it effectively. One of the best ways to possibly escape this terrifying disease appears to be through healthy living, pure and simple.

Part of this lifestyle strategy involves good nutrition, specifically eating a diet high in the B vitamin folate. This nutrient battles the effects of homocysteine in the body, a protein that contributes to clogged arteries and heart trouble. Lots of folate in the diet is believed to guard brain cells from damage by homocysteine—so eat plenty of oranges, orange juice, fortified cereals, and green leafy vegetables. For extra nutritional insurance, take in at least 400 micrograms of folic acid a day, the amount found in most multivitamins.

Multi-Infarct Dementia and Stroke

This common form of dementia is caused by a series of strokes (bleeding or lack of blood supply in the brain) that leave pockets of dead brain cells (infarcts). The accumulated effect of these strokes leads to gradual loss of memory; personality changes; depression; sudden, involuntary laughing or crying; partial paralysis of one side of the body; and other symptoms. Another term for multi-infarct dementia is "vascular dementia." It can co-exist with Alzheimer's disease.

Although irreversible, multi-infarct dementia is largely preventable by taking measures to reduce your risk of stroke, as well as your risk of high blood pressure and atherosclerosis (the narrowing and thickening of arteries), two conditions that can lead to stroke. Anti-stroke measures include controlling your weight, cholesterol, and salt intake; getting regular exercise; quitting smoking; avoiding or decreasing the frequency of situations known to cause stress in your life; and getting regular medical check-ups.

Nutritionally, there is a super-strong connection between diet and stroke prevention. The very best protection against stroke is to eat a diet high in fruits and vegetables. A Harvard study revealed that drinking citrus juices and eating cruciferous vegetables such as broccoli, cauliflower, and Brussels sprouts can reduce your stroke risk by as much as 32 percent. Orange juice reduced risk of a blood clot stroke by 25 percent, says another study.

Why do fruits and vegetables offer such amazing protection? For one thing, they are rich in antioxidants such as vitamin C, found in citrus fruits and vegetables, and beta-carotene and other carotenoids, plentiful in yellow, orange, and red vegetables. Your brain consumes more oxygen than any other organ in your body. Thus, it is highly vulnerable to oxidation, a tissue-damaging process that occurs when oxygen reacts with fat. The by-products of this reaction are disease-causing free radicals.

Fortunately though, oxidation and the free radicals it produces can be neutralized by antioxidants, available from carbohydrates and other foods, supplements, and found naturally in your body.

The best way to increase your supply of brain-protective antioxidants is to eat plenty of fruits and vegetables every day—at least five servings of vegetables and three servings of fruits daily. Include a variety of green, orange, yellow, and purple fruits and vegetables in your diet.

It bears repeating that fruits and vegetables are loaded with folate, which has amazing stroke prevention powers because it prevents the build-up of homocysteine in your body. Homocysteine causes the cells lining arterial walls to deteriorate in three ways. It damages the walls of blood vessels, causing them to constrict; it triggers abnormal blood clotting; and it promotes the build-up of plaque. All these factors conspire to increase your risk of stroke. (High homocysteine levels also deflate your mood and cripple your mental acuity.) The "cure" for elevated homocysteine levels is as easy as eating more folate-rich foods like green leafy vegetables and oranges, drinking orange juice, plus taking supplemental folic acid (400 micrograms a day).

Another stroke-preventive nutrient found in fruits and vegetables is the mineral potassium. Not getting enough potassium in your diet can increase your chance of stroke by 50 percent, according to research. Potassium is plen-

tiful in carbs such as bananas, potatoes, California avo-
cadoes, lima beans, tomato juice, spinach, and orange
juice.

For added protection, be sure to eat carbs high in magnesium, a mineral that is widely distributed in foods.
Swiss researchers discovered in 1999 that foods rich in
magnesium were highly protective against stroke. Magnesium helps regulate blood pressure, maintain normal
function of nerves, and protects blood vessels from damage. Carbs such as green vegetables, wheat germ, soybeans, figs, corn, and apples are packed with magnesium.

Clearly, a lot of what goes wrong with your brain,
though distressing, is eminently preventable or highly
treatable—mostly by adopting healthier lifestyle habits.
Those habits, including a diet filled with good carbs, can
go a long way toward outsmarting problems with your
mind, your mood, and your memory.

FIVE

The Carb-Cancer Connection

If there were ever a case to be made for avoiding bad carbs, their link to cancer would seal it shut. Highly refined carbohydrates such as sugar, white flour, and other bad carbs are tied to an increased risk of at least four types of cancer: breast, colon, lung, and pancreatic. Consider the following evidence.

BREAST CANCER

Several studies conducted in recent years have looked into the link between bad carbs and breast cancer—the second leading cause of cancer death in women after lung cancer. In 2001, Italian researchers reported in the *Annals of Oncology* that high-glycemic index foods such as white bread increased a woman's chances of getting breast cancer by 40 percent, while medium-glycemic index foods like pasta did not affect risk. The researchers based their conclusions on their analysis of nearly 2,500 dietary records of women who had breast cancer.

COLON CANCER

*Studies of large populations have turned up rather con-*sistent findings: that diets high in added, refined sugar are associated with a greater risk of colon cancer, the third most common form of cancer found in men and women in the United States. In a 1997 study, for example, researchers at the University of Utah analyzed the dietary records of nearly 2,000 people and found that those who ate a lot of sugar and simple carbs were at a greater risk than people whose diets were high in healthier, complex carbs. In a similar study, conducted in 2001, Italian researchers looked into the relationship between high-glycemic index diets and cancers of the colon and rectum by calculating the average daily glycemic index and fiber intake of roughly 2,000 people who had filled out food questionnaires. The researchers discovered that the odds of getting either of these cancers went up considerably with a diet that was high in refined carbohydrates.

LUNG CANCER

Lung cancer is the deadliest form of cancer among men and women. More people die annually of this cancer than of colon, breast, and prostate cancers combined. While the greatest lifestyle risk factor for lung cancer is smoking, another might be a high-sugar diet. That's the finding of a study published in *Nutrition and Cancer* in 1998 by a team of researchers from Uruguay. They analyzed the dietary records of 463 people with various types of lung cancer, and after removing smoking and other factors from the research equation, they found that a high intake of sugar was associated with a greater risk of lung cancer.

PANCREATIC CANCER

Pancreatic cancer is the fourth leading cause of cancer death in men and women in the United States. Looking into a link between pancreatic cancer and carbohydrates, a team of researchers from the National Cancer Institute analyzed the dietary records of women participating in the Nurses' Health Study, an ongoing study of the relationship between health habits and disease in nearly 90,000 nurses who have been tracked since 1976. Zeroing in on the women's sugar and carbohydrate intakes, the researchers discovered that sedentary, overweight women who ate meals high in added sugar and white flour (both bad carbs) had a 53 percent increased risk of pancreatic cancer.

UNDERSTANDING THE CARB-CANCER CONNECTION

In these cancers, the major connection to carbohydrates hinges on the carbs ranked as "fast" on the glycemic index scale, one of the scorecards used in chapter 2 to rate carbs. Eating fast carbs makes your glucose and insulin levels go sky high. This in turn might raise levels of "insulinlike growth factors." Insulinlike growth factors are chemicals in the body that might promote cancer when produced in excess by increasing abnormal cell growth that leads to cancer.

Soaring insulin levels, which are the result of a diet too high in refined carbohydrates, can also lead to insulin resistance, a metabolic disturbance that is linked to cancer risk. In insulin resistance, cells don't respond to insulin properly. Because insulin's job is to help your cells use and store glucose from the digestion and absorption of food, cells receive no nourishment and, thereby, run the risk of impaired function.

Beyond the insulin connection, bad carbs are practically devoid of cancer-fighting food components such as antioxidants, phytochemicals, fiber, and many other vital food factors. Take refined flour, for example. It gets stripped of 60 to 90 percent of its critical vitamins and minerals during the milling process.

From another angle, several types of bad-carb junk foods, namely snack chips and french fries, contain alarmingly high levels of a cancer-causing chemical called acrylamide, according to tests commissioned by the Center for Science in the Public Interest (CSPI), as well as studies conducted by the Swedish government. Acrylamide forms as a result of chemical reactions that take place during baking or frying at high temperatures. It is found in high amounts in potato chips, corn chips, frozen french fries, and fast-food french fries. In fact, the amount of acrylamide in a large order of fast-food french fries is around 300 times more than what the U.S. Environmental Protection Agency (EPA) allows in a glass of water! (Acrylamide is sometimes used in water-treatment processes.) Acrylamide is one more reason to avoid bad carbs that contain it.

From a global perspective, the number of new cancer cases is expected to rise by 50 percent over the next 20 years, according to new data from the World Health Organization (WHO). The reason for this increase is because poor nations are adopting bad Western habits, like smoking, drinking, eating the wrong kinds of carbs and other foods, and not exercising. It just so happens that rich nations, like the United States, have higher rates of cancer than poor ones, mostly because of unhealthy lifestyles.

When you consider all the evidence, one thing is clear: If you want to live a lifestyle associated with a low risk of cancer, cutting back on sugar, refined carbohydrates, junk food, and high-glycemic carbohydrates is a powerful change you can make right away.

Although the evidence indicting bad carbs is fairly strong, there is even stronger evidence showing that good carbs, namely fruits, vegetables, and whole grains, are powerful protectors against cancer. In fact, good nutrition is now recognized by scientists and medical experts as playing a major role in slashing the risk of many cancers. The American Institute for Cancer Research (AIRC) estimates that 375,000 cases of cancer could be prevented every year in the United States if we made better dietary choices. Plus, Harvard's School of Public Health suggests that improved diets, more exercise, and other healthy lifestyle habits might help cut cancer deaths by as much as one third. Clearly, there is growing evidence that many good carbs, along with a healthy lifestyle, can help you prevent many different types of cancers. For information on which carbs might prevent certain types of cancer, refer to the following chart.

CANCERS	POTENTIALLY PROTECTIVE GOOD CARBS
Bladder	Garlic, green leafy vegetables, soy foods, yellow/orange vegetables, and yogurt and other fermented milk products
Breast	Apples, bran, beans and legumes, broccoli, Brussels sprouts, button and shiitake mushrooms, cabbage, carrots and carrot juice, cherries, garlic, kohlrabi, low-fat dairy products (with the exception of skim milk), radishes, soy foods, spinach, whole grains, yellow/orange vegetables, and yogurt
Cervical	Romaine lettuce and other green leafy vegetables, tomatoes and tomato products, and yellow/orange vegetables

(continued)

CANCERS	POTENTIALLY PROTECTIVE GOOD CARBS
Colon	Broccoli, Brussels sprouts, cabbage, carrots, cauliflower, celery, garlic, grapes and grape juice, kale, legumes, lettuce, low-fat dairy products, oat bran, oranges and orange juice, spinach, tomatoes and tomato products, wheat bran, whole grains, and yogurt and other fermented milk products
Endometrial	Broccoli, Brussels sprouts, cabbage, cauliflower, kale and other green leafy vegetables, and yellow/orange vegetables
Esophageal	Tomatoes and tomato products
Liver	Garlic
Lung	Broccoli, Brussels sprouts, cabbage, carrots and other yellow/orange vegetables, cauliflower, hot peppers, kale, onions, oranges, spinach and other green leafy vegetables, and tomatoes and tomato products
Oral	Tomatoes and tomato products
Ovarian	Broccoli, Brussels sprouts, cabbage, cauliflower, kale and other green leafy vegetables, and yellow/orange vegetables
Pancreatic	Legumes and tomatoes and tomato products
Prostate	Brussels sprouts, broccoli, cabbage, canola oil, cauliflower, kale, low-fat dairy products, soy foods, and tomatoes and tomato products
Stomach	Broccoli, Brussels sprouts, cabbage, cauliflower, fava beans, garlic, green tea, kale, onions, oranges and other citrus fruits, tomatoes and tomato products, and whole grains

CANCER-FIGHTING CARBS

Eat more good carbs and you'll become healthier—and perhaps free of cancer. This message is coming through loud and clear from research studies, major medical organizations, physicians, cancer specialists, and many other sources. But to make the right dietary adjustments, you need to know which cancer-fighting nutrients are found in which carbs. Here is a rundown.

Antioxidants

As you will recall, antioxidants are vitamins and minerals that protect the body against disease-causing free radicals. To foil these cellular terrorists, antioxidants step in, scour them from the body, and prevent new ones from being formed. Where cancer is concerned, three of the main antioxidants are vitamin C, vitamin E, and selenium—all plentiful in good carbs such as fruits, vegetables, and whole grains. Here's a closer look.

Vitamin C

There's plenty of evidence linking vitamin C to the prevention of cancer. More than a dozen studies have shown that vitamin C, a powerful antioxidant, reduces the risk of almost all forms of cancer, including cancers of the bladder, breast, cervix, colon, esophagus, larynx, lung, mouth, prostate, pancreas, and stomach. Best news of all: Most of the evidence for this anticancer benefit comes from studies of high vitamin C intake from foods, not from supplements!

As a cancer fighter, vitamin C appears to work in a couple important ways. It disarms free radicals before they can damage DNA (which controls cell growth and reproduction) and stimulate tumor growth. It assists the body's own free-radical defense mechanism by working in partnership with vitamin E to arrest free radicals.

The best sources of vitamin C in the diet are good carbs such as citrus fruits. Other foods, such as green and red peppers, collard greens, broccoli, Brussels sprouts, cabbage, spinach, cantaloupe, and strawberries are also excellent sources, and you should try to eat a variety of these foods. In addition, there are other ways to get more vitamin C in your diet:

- Eat at least one citrus fruit daily. Oranges are an exceptional choice because they contain flavonoids (see below) that enhance the absorption of vitamin C.

- Take in extra vitamin C by drinking citrus juice rather than sodas.

- Eat fresh, raw sources of vitamin C whenever possible. Cooking destroys much of the vitamin C in foods.

Vitamin E

Vitamin E is emerging as an important nutrient for fighting one type of cancer: colon. In a five-year study of more than 35,000 women, researchers observed that those who developed colon cancer were the same ones who had low dietary intakes of vitamin E, according to food questionnaires that were filled out and analyzed. The researchers speculated that vitamin E protected cell membranes in the colon against destruction that could lead to cancer.

Vitamin E also inhibits the formation of carcinogenic substances known as "nitrosamines," which are formed from chemicals called nitrates and nitrites, sometimes found in processed meats like hot dogs and salami. Nitrosamines have been implicated in the development of stomach cancer.

Vitamin E is a fat-soluble vitamin, meaning that it can be stored with fat in the liver and other tissues. Vitamin E is also a component of cells, sandwiched between the fatty layers that make up cell membranes. When free radicals come along, they hitch up to vitamin E, damaging it instead of the rest of the cell membrane. In the process, vitamin E soaks up the free radicals, and the cell is protected from damage. Of all antioxidant nutrients, vitamin E does the best job of scavenging free radicals.

Vitamin E is found widely in foods, particularly vegetable oils. One important carb source of vitamin E is wheat germ. Fruits and vegetables also supply appreciable amounts. To increase your vitamin E intake from natural carb sources:

- Sprinkle wheat germ on your cereal in the morning, or mix wheat germ with yogurt.

- Eat an apple a day (apples contain vitamin E).

- Use dried black currants in lieu of raisins, because currants contain vitamin E.

- Stick to vitamin E–rich whole grains such as wheat, rice, oats, rye, and barley, rather than refined grain products, because vitamin E is removed in the milling process.

Selenium

Among the chief antioxidant minerals is selenium. It works by producing glutathione peroxidase, an antioxidant enzyme that can turn troublesome free radicals into harmless water. This mineral also works closely with vitamin E in protecting the body against free radicals.

The mineral might be an important safeguard against cancer. Studies have found that people with high levels of selenium have lower rates of skin cancer, prostate cancer, colon cancer, and lung cancer.

Selenium is plentiful in carbs such as whole grains and legumes. To get more selenium-rich carbs in your diet:

* Go meatless several times a week by serving bean- and legume-based dishes.

* Opt for whole grains over refined cereals. (Selenium is another nutrient removed during the milling process.)

* Select high-selenium foods. Some of the best vegetable sources include onions and broccoli.

* Cook with garlic, another good source of selenium.

Phytoestrogens

Tofu and other soy-based carbs are loaded with natural, hormonally active compounds called phytoestrogens. These substances attach themselves to cancer cells and prevent real estrogen from entering the cells and allowing cancer to grow. Phytoestrogens also act as antioxidants that have been shown to fight free-radical damage that can lead to cancer.

Evidence of the power of phytoestrogens can be seen among people who eat a lot of soy foods. Asian women, for example, eat low-fat diets with large amounts of tofu and other soy-based products. They have five times less the rate of breast cancer than women who eat a typical Western diet. When breast cancer does strike Asian women, it takes a more favorable course and has a higher cure rate.

Men shouldn't feel left out. Because of their regulating action on hormones, phytoestrogens might help prevent prostate cancer, another hormone-dependent cancer. Scientists also feel that phytoestrogens in soy foods might directly inhibit the growth and spread of hormone-needy cancer cells. In fact, soy consumption is proving to be more protective against prostate cancer than any other dietary factor, according to a prostate cancer mortality study conducted in forty-two countries. In test tubes, soy protein actually kills off prostate cancer cells.

A good move is to include more soy products in your diet, particularly as substitutes for meat or milk in low-fat cooking. Here are some suggestions for sneaking more phytoestrogens into your diet:

- Select foods that are highest in phytoestrogens. Some of the best sources are soybeans and soybean products.

- Use soy milk on your cereal and blend into smoothies.

- Try soy burgers in place of hamburgers.

- Use textured soy protein in recipes calling for ground beef.

- Snack on soy-based nutrition bars rather than on candy bars.

- Use tofu on crackers and rice cakes and in Italian recipes like lasagna to replace all or part of the ricotta cheese. Tofu can also be blended into shakes and smoothies, plus used as a base for dips.

- Munch on soy nuts or soy chips, available at most health food stores.

- Replace some of the flour in recipes with soy flour.

Flavonoids

Packing a wallop of power against cancer are a group of natural substances called flavonoids, found abundantly in fruits, vegetables, and whole grains. More than 5,000 flavonoids have been discovered in nature, and many are responsible for the bright colors of the fruits and vegetables you eat. Flavonoids are also essential for the proper

absorption of vitamin C, one of the most important antioxidants and cancer fighters. In fact, flavonoids are what
make natural vitamin C (found in foods) more effective
than synthetic supplemental vitamin C by improving and
prolonging the function of the vitamin. Flavonoids and
other beneficial plant compounds might be the reason why
women who eat lots of fruits, vegetables, and whole
grains have far fewer cases of breast cancer.

Some of the more familiar flavonoids are catechins, ci-
trin, hesperidin, quercetin, and rutin. Of these, catechins
and quercetin have been the best studied for their protection against cancer.

Catechins are abundant in green and black teas, red
wine, and chocolate. Research with animals shows that
catechins inhibit cancers of most major organs: skin, lung,
esophagus, stomach, liver, small intestine, colon, pancreas, bladder, and mammary gland.

Quercetin is among the top flavonoids in our diets,
present in fruits, vegetables, and tea. As noted earlier, research shows that quercetin is protective against prostate
cancer, lung cancer, and skin cancer.

Scientists believe that quercetin, catechins, and other
flavonoids exert their anticancer effect in three possible
ways. First, they act as antioxidants, squelching free radicals. Second, flavonoids appear to interfere with the
growth and spread of tumors, possibly by inhibiting "tumor angiogenesis." This is an abnormal process by which
new blood vessels are formed to feed tumors. When these
supply routes are cut off, tumors can't get the oxygen and
nutrients they need to grow. And third, flavonoids fight
cancer by increasing the ability of cells to flush out carcinogens.

All fruits and vegetables are well endowed with a variety of cancer-fighting flavonoids. Here are some other
ways to increase flavonoid-rich carbs into your diet:

- Season your foods with chopped garlic or onion.

- Eat a salad every day.

- Eat a variety of fruits and vegetables.

- Try a new fruit or vegetable every week.

- Include at least two vegetables with lunch and dinner.

- Double your portion of vegetables at lunch or dinner.

- Top your breakfast cereal with fresh berries.

- Add extra vegetables to soups and stews.

- Go meatless several times a week.

- Eat vegetable burgers, rather than hamburgers, more frequently.

Carotenoids

Don't risk cancer by shortchanging yourself on orange, red, and yellow fruits and vegetables. As mentioned previously, these good carbs are loaded with carotenoids. Beta-carotene, the best known of the carotenoids, might reduce the risk of cancers of the colon, rectum, breast, uterus, and prostate.

Other important carotenoids include alpha-carotene, shown to protect against breast cancer; beta-cryptoxanthin, which looks promising against breast cancer and lung cancer; lutein, which might guard against cancer of the colon, lung, and breast; lycopene, which appears to be protective against cancer of the prostate, colon, bladder, and pancreas; and zeaxanthin, which is linked to a lower risk of breast, cervical, and colon cancers.

Here are some tips for super-charging your diet with carotenoids:

- Fill your plate with as many colorful vegetables as you can. The more colorful your food selections, the more carotenoids you'll eat.

- Eat canned soups with a tomato base.

- Add a jar or two of strained carrots (yes—baby food!) to soups or stews; it is loaded with carotenoids.

- Drink vegetable juices rather than sodas.

- Eat a hefty serving of tomatoes or tomato-based foods at least twice a week or more.

- Add extra tomato sauce or paste to soups or stews.

- Eat sandwiches and salads with tomatoes.

- Snack on raw fruits and vegetables to get the most carotenoids. One exception, though, is carrots, which actually release more carotenoids when cooked.

- Enjoy exotic fruits such as guavas or mangoes for a change of pace.

- Blend cooked carrots or pumpkin into a smoothie.

Folate

Folate, a member of the B-complex family of vitamins, is critical for the synthesis, repair, and functioning of DNA, the genetic material of cells. In fact, numerous scientific experiments have revealed that folate deficiencies cause DNA damage that resembles the DNA damage in cancer cells. This finding has led scientists to suggest that cancer could be initiated by DNA damage caused by a deficiency in this B-complex vitamin.

Research shows that folate suppresses cell growth in colon cancer. It also prevents the formation of precancerous lesions that could lead to cervical cancer—a discovery that might explain why women who do not eat many vegetables and fruits (good sources of folate) have higher rates of this form of cancer. Other studies link low intake of folate to an increased risk of breast, lung, uterine, and pancreatic cancers.

Folate is found in a wide variety of foods, mainly vegetables, cereals, and grains. To get more of this amazing nutrient in your diet:

• Prepare salads using the darkest-leaf lettuce possible (such as romaine). These varieties are higher in folate.

• Incorporate spinach and other green leafy vegetables into recipes such as those for soups, lasagna, and casseroles.

• Drink a glass of orange juice most days of the week. It's loaded with folate.

• Switch to folate-fortified cereals.

Fiber

Every time you bite into a juicy apple, you're eating fiber, an indigestible but indispensable part of food. An ever-growing body of research suggests that you can reduce your odds of getting cancer by increasing your fiber intake to the recommend level of 25 to 35 grams a day. Studies have found that eating more fiber:

• Might reduce the risk of colon cancer by up to 40 percent.

• Lowers the risk of stomach cancer by 60 percent, especially if that fiber is cereal fiber.

• Cuts your risk of cancers of the mouth and throat by half.

How exactly does fiber fight cancer? It does so by detoxifying and eliminating harmful dietary factors and carcinogens from your body. One type of carcinogen eradicated from the body by fiber is bile acid, a by-product of fat digestion. Increased levels of bile acid in the stool can cause cells in the mucous membranes of the intestines to grow abnormally and possibly lead to colon cancer.

Fiber also eliminates hormonal by-products (including estrogen) made by your body that can lead to breast cancer. Normally, these hormonal by-products are excreted in your bowel, but if you shortchange yourself with too little fiber in your diet, food will take days to travel from entry to exit, creating chronic constipation. With constipation, these by-products remain in your system and are reabsorbed back into your body. So by preventing constipation, fiber might indirectly prevent breast cancer. But not only breast cancer: Regularity is important in preventing stomach, pancreatic, and prostate cancer. So making sure there's plenty of fiber in your diet is an excellent way to prevent constipation and, thus, keep cancer-causing by-products moving naturally out of your body.

The key is to populate your diet with more high-fiber foods. Some of your best fiber bets include vegetables, fruits, cereals, and whole grains. To pump up your fiber intake:

- Eat a wide variety of natural foods in reasonable amounts. (There are at least six different types of fiber in foods, and all are vital to good health. By varying your food selections, you ensure that you also eat a variety of these important fibers.)

- Eat a large salad most days of the week. Choose darker-leaf lettuces; they're higher in fiber and other nutrients.

- Eat fruits and vegetables raw and unpeeled whenever possible. (They have far more fiber than foods that have been peeled, cooked, and otherwise processed.)

- Choose whole-grain cereals such as oatmeal, oat bran, bulgur wheat, and brown rice throughout the week.

- Select dry, unsweetened cereals to which extra fiber has been purposely added as part of the product formulation.

- Add high-fiber grains such as barley or brown rice to vegetable soups.

- Sprinkle raw wheat bran over cereals and salads. In research, bran has been shown to reduce levels of hormonal by-products and other potential carcinogens.

- Substitute high-fiber foods such as beans and lentils for meat and poultry several times a week.

Good carbs, the ones that have been listed and discussed so far in this book, are loaded with protective factors that pay big dividends when it comes to fighting cancer. Variety is the key. When you eat a wide range of fruits, vegetables, and whole grains, you are supplying your body with the full armor of protection against this deadly disease.

SIX

The Diabetes Defense

For preventing and treating diabetes and other blood sugar disorders, carbohydrates are the most important food group because they have the most pronounced effect on your blood sugar levels. After you eat carbohydrates, your blood sugar rises, and insulin is secreted in response. Insulin's job is to keep your blood sugar within normal ranges—neither too high nor too low—by shuttling that blood sugar into your cells for energy, thereby lowering levels of glucose in your blood.

Sometimes though, normal insulin activity is upset, and cells cannot use glucose properly. This results in either type I diabetes or type II diabetes, two of the most common blood-sugar-related medical problems. Though treatable, diabetes is the seventh leading cause of death in the United States, and 16 million people have it.

In type I diabetes, the body does not produce any insulin, and consequently, cells cannot absorb glucose. Type I diabetic patients, who typically get the disease at a young age, must, therefore, rely on daily injections of insulin to survive. You're at a greater risk of developing type I diabetes if your siblings or parents have the disease.

Type II diabetes is the most common form of the disease, accounting for 90 to 95 percent of all cases. In type II diabetes, the body can't make enough insulin or use it properly. Consequently, glucose does not get into cells as it should, and there is a glut of glucose in the blood.

Risk factors for type II diabetes are linked largely to age and lifestyle factors, although genetic factors are involved, too. With age, for example, your body gradually loses its ability to regulate glucose. This puts you in danger of developing the disease, which can typically occur in people over 45 years old, particularly among those who are overweight. In fact, more than 80 percent of type II diabetics are overweight. What's more, type II diabetes is present in 25 percent of the population age 85 and older.

Diabetes has been dubbed the "silent killer" because most people are unaware that they have it until diagnosed with one of its life-threatening complications, such as blindness, kidney disease, nerve disease, or cardiovascular disease. In fact, the American Diabetes Association estimates that there are 5.4 million people in the United States who have diabetes but don't know it. There are some warning signs, however, and these are listed in the following table.

WARNING SIGNS OF DIABETES

Type I Diabetes	*Type II Diabetes
• Frequent urination • Increased thirst • Increased appetite • Unexplained weight loss • Extreme fatigue • Irritability	• Any of the type I symptoms • Frequent infections • Blurred vision • Slow-healing wounds • Tingling or numbness in hands or feet • Recurring skin, gum, or bladder infections

*Often, people with type II diabetes experience no symptoms.

Source: American Diabetes Association

DIET AND DIABETES

The primary treatment for type I diabetes is insulin, taken by injection. Type II diabetes, on the other hand, can be managed by changes in diet and exercise and often by drugs other than insulin.

If you have either form of diabetes, food is one of the chief tools you can use to control the disease and stay healthy. Food helps keep your blood sugar in line, provides energy for exercise and daily activities, and supplies the nutrients needed for health and healing. Food is nourishment and medicine all rolled into one.

What kind of food should you eat if you have diabetes? A prevailing myth about diabetes is that you must follow a special "diabetic diet." Not so. You have the same nutritional needs as anyone else. Like the rest of the world, you need regular, well-balanced meals that provide a variety of nutrients from carbohydrates, protein, and fat.

Here is an overview of what you need if you have diabetes:

Carbohydrates. Roughly half of your diet (40 to 50 percent of your total daily calories) should be made up of carbohydrates, with an emphasis on natural, high-fiber choices, such as vegetables, legumes, fruits, and whole grains. Because carbohydrates are so important in diabetes, they will be discussed in detail later in the chapter.

Protein. Protein intake should make up 10 to 20 percent of your total daily calories. Choose lean, low-fat proteins from poultry, fish, dairy, and vegetable sources such as beans, legumes, and tofu. (If you have kidney disease—often a complication of diabetes—you might be placed on a protein-restricted diet, because excess protein places an undue burden on the kidneys. Your doctor will probably recommend that you reduce your protein intake to around 10 percent of your daily calories.)

Fat. Generally, a healthy intake of fat is 30 percent or less of your total daily calories. Less than 10 percent should come from saturated fats (fats that are solid at room temperature). The remaining 10 to 15 percent should come from polyunsaturated fats (available from fish and vegetable oils) and monounsaturated fats (found in olive oil and nuts). Dietary cholesterol should be limited to less than 300 milligrams daily to discourage cardiovascular disease, which is the major complication of diabetes. Cholesterol is found in eggs, meats, and high-fat dairy products.

GOOD CARBS AND DIABETES

Ideally, in a diet to control diabetes you should use all three carbohydrate scorecards to select only the healthiest carbs for your diet. For example:

Simple versus complex. Most of the carbohydrates in

your diet should come from the good carbs such as complex carbohydrates. These carbs furnish more vitamins, minerals, antioxidants, and phytochemicals than simple carbohydrates do.

Sugar, a simple carbohydrate, is no longer a forbidden food in diabetes. It is perfectly fine to include a little bit of sugar and sugar-containing foods in your diet, and you don't really have to avoid table sugar, corn sweeteners, syrups, or other such foods. Eating sugar and sugar-containing foods does not hurt blood-sugar control in either type I or type II diabetes. However, you should not go overboard, because sugar is a poor nutritional choice and is tied to heart disease, obesity, and cancer. If you wish to restrict sugar but have a bit of a sweet tooth, opt for artificial sweeteners instead.

Fast versus slow (glycemic index). You can use the glycemic index to select carbohydrates that are less likely to cause roller-coaster swings in your blood sugar. There are benefits to doing so. Research has found that following low-glycemic index diets, on average, can lower your blood glucose and insulin by as much as 30 percent. Because low-GI foods have appetite-control and fat-burning benefits, incorporating them into your diet can help you shed pounds.

Low fiber versus high fiber. The carbohydrates you choose should be rich in fiber because of its beneficial effects on glucose and insulin metabolism. High-fiber foods require prolonged breakdown and, thus, release blood sugar more slowly. This action helps prevent dips in blood sugar and helps maintain even energy levels throughout the day. A study published recently in the *New England Journal of Medicine* reported that people with type II diabetes could lower their blood sugar and insulin levels by as much as 10 percent simply by eating a fiber-rich diet.

The type of fiber most responsible for this glucose-lowering effect is soluble fiber, found in oat bran, oatmeal, barley, peas, beans, carrots, apples, and oranges.

Try to shoot for 25 to 35 grams of fiber a day from fruits, vegetables, beans, and whole grains.

The following chart lists good carbs that should be included in your diet most days of the week.

TOP 15 ANTIDIABETIC CARBS

Carbohydrate	Beneficial Action
Apples	High in the soluble fiber pectin, which helps control blood sugar; also high in beneficial plant compounds called flavonoids, which help prevent diabetic complications.
Barley, pearled	High in the soluble fiber pectin, which helps control blood sugar; also a low-GI food.
Broccoli	Contains glutathione, an antioxidant that helps reduce the risk of diabetes and its complications.
Brown rice	High in the mineral chromium, which helps regulate blood sugar.
Carrots	Although higher on the glycemic index, carrots contain beneficial substances called carotenoids (beta-carotene is a carotenoid) that might protect against abnormal elevations in blood sugar.
Garlic	Contains a beneficial plant compound called allicin, which helps lower blood sugar.
Green leafy vegetables	Rich in antioxidants and phytochemicals, which help prevent diabetic complications.
Jerusalem artichokes	Contain a beneficial substance called inulin, which helps lower blood sugar after a meal, probably by slowing its absorption in the intestine.

(continued)

TOP 15 ANTIDIABETIC CARBS

Carbohydrate	Beneficial Action
Kidney beans	Among beans and legumes, the kidney bean is the highest in soluble fiber, which reduces the rise in blood sugar after a meal, normalizes insulin levels, and helps keep blood sugar levels steady throughout the day.
Oat bran	High in the soluble fiber pectin, which helps control blood sugar.
Onions	High in beneficial plant compounds called flavonoids, which help prevent diabetic complications.
Pumpkin	Contains beneficial substances called carotenoids (beta-carotene is a carotenoid) that might protect against abnormal elevations in blood sugar. Although higher on the glycemic index, pumpkin is rich in fiber.
Rye bread	Enhances insulin secretion in the pancreas, where insulin is produced.
Soybeans	High in fiber; also high in biotin, a B vitamin that enhances the body's use of insulin and is beneficial in the regulation of blood sugar.
Whole grains	High in fiber; also beneficial in helping the body use insulin; lowers the risk of type II diabetes.

WORKING WITH CARBOHYDRATES IN YOUR DIET

If you have diabetes, your meal planning should focus on low-fat nutrition, moderate amounts of protein, and designated quantities of high-fiber, complex carbohydrates, with priority given to the amount of carbohydrates you eat. Your diet should also be consistent; that is, you should eat roughly the same amount of calories each day, eat meals and snacks at the same time every day, and not miss meals. In addition, structure your meals to include a variety of many different types of foods.

A meal planning system growing in favor for managing diabetes is "carbohydrate counting." This is a method of counting the grams of carbohydrates you eat at meals and snacks. The reason for counting carbohydrates is because they have the most dramatic effect on your glucose levels. Your body converts carbohydrates into glucose faster than it does protein or fat. In fact, carbohydrate is converted to glucose within the first two hours after you eat a meal.

If you know how much carbohydrate you've eaten, you can predict what your blood glucose will do. A little bit of carbohydrates will elevate your glucose, and large amounts will make it go up even higher. For example, a full cup of cereal will make your blood glucose go higher than a half-cup, and two cups will elevate it even more.

These metabolic facts of life have particular importance if you take insulin, which is required to balance the glucose. It is the amount of carbohydrates in a meal that largely determines how much insulin you require. Counting carbohydrates, therefore, can help you make appropriate insulin adjustments based on your blood glucose patterns.

With this method of meal planning, carbohydrates are computed in grams and usually translated into "carbohydrate choices." For example, 1 carbohydrate choice = 15 grams of carbohydrate. You can find information on how much carbohydrate is in foods by checking the Nutrition Facts Panel on food labels, or by consulting a carbohydrate gram counter guide.

Carbohydrate counting has been found to be among the

most effective tools ever devised for controlling blood sugar and achieving other treatment goals. It works best if you:

- Need to prevent swings in your blood sugar.

- Want to eat the same amount of carbohydrates at given times to help stabilize your levels of blood glucose.

- Are within a reasonable body weight range.

- Have type I diabetes and need to better match your insulin to the foods you eat.

- Are willing to monitor your blood glucose levels before and after meals and keep records of the results.

- Have had an inconsistent carbohydrate intake in the past.

- Have been unsuccessful using other meal-planning systems.

- Have been newly diagnosed with diabetes.

- Have had diabetes for a long time and are willing to try a new approach to meal planning.

- Like to work with numbers.

HOW TO PLAN A CARBOHYDRATE COUNTING DIET

Again, carbohydrates should make up roughly one-half of your required calories. With carbohydrate counting, carbohydrates are divided equally into meals and snacks. Eating the same quantity of carbohydrates at each meal helps stabilize blood glucose levels.

Thus, you build your daily meals and snacks around a

fairly consistent number of carbohydrate grams, which translate into carbohydrate choices. In addition to carbohydrate choices, you'll also choose protein foods and fats. Here is an example of a daily diet planned by using this system.

CARBOHYDRATE COUNTING: SAMPLE MEAL PLAN

Meals and Snacks	Carbohydrate Grams	Carbohydrate Choices	Foods
Breakfast	60 grams of carbohydrate	4 carbohydrate choices	½ cup oatmeal, or 1 banana (small), or 1 large bran muffin (counts as 2 carbohydrate choices)
	1 ounce of protein	1 ounce of protein	1 hard-boiled egg
	2 fats	2 fats	2 teaspoons butter or margarine
Lunch	60 grams of carbohydrate	4 carbohydrate choices	1 whole-grain hamburger bun (counts as 2 carbohydrate choices), or lettuce and tomato slices, or low-fat yogurt sweetened with aspartame, or 1 cup raspberries
	3 ounces of protein	3 ounces of protein	3-ounce hamburger patty
	1 fat	1 fat	1 teaspoon mayonnaise
Dinner	60 grams of carbohydrate	4 carbohydrate choices	Salad (1 cup greens; or 1 cup chopped raw salad veggies, or and ½ cup artichoke hearts); or 1 baked potato; or 1 roll; or ½ cup water-packed fruit cocktail

(continued)

CARBOHYDRATE COUNTING: SAMPLE MEAL PLAN

Meals and Snacks	Carbohydrate Grams	Carbohydrate Choices	Foods
Dinner	3 ounces of protein 2 fats	3 ounces of protein 2 fats	3 ounces grilled salmon 2 teaspoons French salad dressing
Snack	30 grams of carbohydrates	2 carbohydrate choices	3 whole-wheat crackers; or 1 cup skim milk

Nutrition: Approximately 1,800 calories; 53 percent of calories from carbohydrates; 21 percent of calories from protein; 26 percent of calories from fat; 25 grams of fiber.

Adapted from: Benedict, M. "Carbohydrate counting: tips for simplifying diabetes education." Health Care Food and Nutrition Focus, 16: 6–9, 1999; and Greenwood-Robinson, M. Control Diabetes in Six Easy Steps, 2002.

If you are interested in learning more about carbohydrate counting, work with a registered dietitian who is well versed in the system. Your dietitian will help you master the system; identify patterns of blood sugar levels that are related to your diet, diabetes medications, and physical activity; and teach you how to calculate the amount of insulin you need to control blood sugar when you eat a specific amount of carbohydrate.

At the same time, educate yourself on how many grams of carbohydrates are in the foods you eat. Initially, you'll have to weigh and measure your foods, but with time, you'll be able to eyeball the correct portions.

USING SPECIAL DIABETIC SUPPLEMENTS

*Although it is generally best to get your good carbs di-*rectly from food, you can get a little more of a good thing through diabetic supplements, specially formulated to help you control your blood sugar. For example:

Diabetic Snack Bars

What they are: Diabetic snack bars are designed to prevent hypoglycemia, a lower-than-normal concentration of glucose in the blood, or reduce hyperglycemia, abnormally high levels of glucose in the blood. These products can be used as convenient snacks or as an occasional meal replacement if you have diabetes.

How they work: Diabetic snack bars contain special carbohydrates that result in better-controlled blood sugar levels. Some products are formulated with uncooked cornstarch, a slowly absorbed complex carbohydrate that provides a sustained source of glucose. Examples of products containing uncooked cornstarch include Extend Bar, Nite Bite, and Gluc-O-Bar. Studies show that bars containing uncooked cornstarch do an excellent job of preventing low blood sugar. In a clinical trial involving the Extend Bar, the product helped ward off low blood sugar for up to nine hours in diabetic patients.

Other diabetic snack bars contain a special kind of carbohydrate called "resistant starch," which is broken down into glucose more slowly than other carbohydrates. In contrast to uncooked cornstarch, which is slowly but fully digested in the small intestine, resistant starch is not completely digested and is, thus, lower in calories. Bars with resistant starch have been proven in research to stabilize blood sugar levels, preventing abnormal and potentially dangerous spikes in glucose. Examples of products with resistant starch are Choice dm (Mead Johnson Nutritionals) and Glucerna (Abbott Laboratories).

How to use them: Diabetic snack bars with uncooked cornstarch are designed to be used as a bedtime snack because they prevent episodes of hypoglycemia that can sometimes occur overnight (a condition called "nocturnal hypoglycemia"). Bars with resistant starch are meant to help prevent elevations in blood sugar during the day.

Safety: Diabetic snack bars are safe when used as directed and as part of an overall nutritional and medical strategy for managing diabetes.

Diabetic Beverages

What they are: Diabetic beverages are a special type of liquid carbohydrate supplement, that like diabetic snack bars, are formulated for people with diabetes. The two leading products, available in pharmacies and grocery stores, are Choice dm beverages and Ensure Glucerna beverages. Both are available in ready-to-drink cans.

How they work: Most of these beverages are rich in slowly digested complex carbohydrates, protein, fiber, contain little or no fat, and are fortified with vitamins and minerals. They provide therapeutic support to help control blood sugar, particularly in conjunction with diabetes drugs, and are geared toward helping reduce the complications of diabetes. Tested clinically, these products help stabilize blood sugar.

How to use them: Diabetic beverages are meant to be used as a snack or as part of a small meal when eaten with fruit or vegetables.

Safety: These products are safe and nutritious when used as directed.

NUTRITIONAL GOALS IN TYPE I DIABETES AND TYPE II DIABETES

With type I or type II diabetes, strive to keep your blood glucose level as close to normal as possible by paying attention to your diet. Here's a summary of the key nutritional goals for each form of diabetes.

If you have type I diabetes:

+ Normalize your blood glucose level through healthy food choices and good meal planning. With tighter glucose control, you'll feel better and lower your odds of getting eye, kidney, or heart disease.

+ Integrate insulin therapy into your eating and exercise patterns.

+ Focus on eating the same amount of carbohydrates at the same meal each day. Select good carbs for your diet.

+ Monitor glucose levels and adjust insulin doses for the amount of food you eat.

+ Plan meals and snacks to prevent hypoglycemia. Consider using diabetic snack bars or beverages.

+ Through diet, exercise, and other lifestyle changes, keep your blood fats (cholesterol and triglycerides) in normal ranges to lower your risk of heart disease. Monitor these levels with regular medical check-ups.

+ Improve your overall health through good nutrition.

If you have type II diabetes:

+ Normalize your blood glucose level, cholesterol, and blood pressure through healthy food choices, good meal planning, and regular medical check-ups.

+ Lose weight if you need to.

+ Plan meals and snacks to prevent hypoglycemia. Consider using diabetic snack bars and beverages as part of your meal planning.

+ Improve your overall diet through the selection of good carbs.

PREVENTING DIABETES

Type I diabetes is primarily a genetic disease, so if it runs in your family, it might be difficult to prevent. Type II diabetes is a different story, however. Although there is a genetic component to type II diabetes, the wonderful news is that you can prevent it with a lifestyle fix that includes mostly diet, exercise, and other nondrug measures. For example:

+ **Good carb nutrition.** Follow a diet that focuses on low-fat nutrition, moderate amounts of lean protein, and good carbs. In planning a preventive diet, 40 to 50 percent of your total daily calories should come from good carbs.

+ **Weight loss and control.** Obesity is a major risk factor for type II diabetes. If you are overweight, begin a sensible reducing diet (see chapter 9 for guidelines on weight control) that is low in fat, high in fiber, and moderate in good carbs. It is best to restrict all bad carbs as much as possible.

+ **Exercise.** Leading an inactive lifestyle contributes to type II diabetes and expedites its progression in two likely ways. First, inactivity leads to obesity, which is the major promoter of type II diabetes. Second, inactivity makes body cells resistant to using insulin and taking in glucose. To overcome these damaging factors, exercise with a program that includes both weight training and aerobics. These activities stimulate normal insulin activity, help your cells take in glucose, and assist you in burning body fat.

• **Quit smoking.** Nicotine harms the ability of your cells to properly respond to and use insulin. Smoking also generates free radicals, which can do irreparable harm to your body.

Many of these same measures can help you prevent, or manage, a condition called "metabolic syndrome" or "syndrome X," which sets the stage for both type II diabetes and cardiovascular disease. The core problem in metabolic syndrome has to do with insulin. If you have metabolic syndrome, your cells defy the action of insulin (insulin resistance), and as a consequence, blood sugar is locked out of cells. Your cells receive little energy or nourishment, and blood sugar piles up in your bloodstream, creating a toxic metabolic environment.

Red flags for this syndrome are knowable through medical testing and include:

• High blood pressure (greater than 130/85; 50 percent of people with high blood pressure have metabolic syndrome)

• Elevated triglycerides (150 or higher)

• Abnormally low HDL cholesterol (less than 50 for women; less than 40 for men)

• Above-normal blood sugar (higher than 110)

• Central obesity, in which your waist measurement is greater than 35 inches if you are a woman and greater than 40 inches if you are a man

Generally, if you have three or more of the above symptoms, your doctor might diagnose you as having metabolic syndrome.

But how does metabolic syndrome develop in the first place? As it turns out, diet is mostly to blame, particularly a diet that's high in bad carbs such as sweets, breads, and processed snack foods. Such foods trigger a rapid spike in blood sugar, and the body responds by pumping out more insulin into the bloodstream to handle the sugar. Over time, insulin levels in your blood remain higher than they should be. This promotes fat storage, elevates blood fats, and raises blood pressure.

Happily though, metabolic syndrome can be prevented and reversed with weight loss, regular exercise, low-fat foods, and a switch from refined carbs to mostly good carbs.

Diabetes might not be curable, but it is manageable and it is preventable. Through proper diet, exercise, and consistent self-care, you can successfully control your diabetes if you have it, and fight it off if you don't. What's more, the sooner you start changing your lifestyle to become more nutritionally and physically fit, the greater your chances of living a full, vigorous, and healthy life.

SEVEN

Digestive Health

•

If your doctor could write you a prescription for pre-
venting a lot of the digestive ills facing mankind, that
prescription would be, in a word, fiber. And you don't
have to go to a pharmacy to get it filled, either. Just eat
a variety of fruits, vegetables, cereals, whole grains, and
other good carbs, and you'll be doing your digestive system a world of good.

Your digestive system is actually a 30-foot long tube,
with an entry at your mouth and an exit at your anus. This
system is supported by other organs, including the liver
and pancreas, which furnish enzymes and other substances
required for digestion. There is a lot that can go right or
wrong along the way, but eating foods rich in fiber is one
important measure you can take to keep this system in
peak health. Fiber prevents, or reduces symptoms of, a
wide range of digestive problems, from appendicitis to
ulcers.

APPENDICITIS

The appendix is a wormlike structure about three inches long that is attached to your colon (also referred to as the large intestine). Until recently, the appendix was believed to have no known function, described by evolutionists as a remnant from the days when man's theorized ancestors (apes) were plant-eaters. In apes and other plant-eating animals, the appendix aids in the digestion of plant material.

New medical evidence, however, has found that the human appendix is indeed a critical organ—one that is an integral part of the disease-fighting immune system. The appendix contains lymphatic tissue whose task it is to attack disease-causing organisms in the lower end of the digestive tract.

Thus, your appendix might protect you from serious illness. A study conducted at a German medical center in 1979 found a higher incidence of ovarian cancer among women who had had their appendix removed (appendectomy). Other medical research has linked appendectomies to an increased susceptibility to leukemia, Hodgkin's disease, and colon cancer.

Based on this medical evidence, it is vital that you do what you can to prevent "appendicitis," an inflammation and infection of the appendix. This is an extremely serious condition in which the appendix can burst if it isn't surgically removed, spreading infection (peritonitis) throughout the abdomen.

Eating a high-fiber diet has been proposed as a way to prevent appendicitis. This recommendation stems from studies of populations of people around the world who eat high-fiber or low-fiber diets. In countries where the diet is mostly grain- and vegetable-based (high-fiber diets), people rarely get appendicitis. By contrast, people who eat low-fiber diets with lots of refined carbohydrates—the typical Western diet—tend to have a higher rates of this disease. Why this occurs is unknown, but some scientists believe that lack of fiber slows down the movement of stools, causing pressure to build and forcing fecal matter into the appendix. Once trapped in the appendix, this material begins to undergo fermentation by natural microbes—a process that produces irritating by-products that might provoke an infection.

In the 2002 issue of the medical journal *Gut,* physician Dr. J. Black recounted a personal World War II story that lends support to the appendicitis-fiber connection. At the end of the war, Dr. Black was stationed at a hospital in South Burma, where nearly 1,100 Japanese soldiers were encamped while awaiting repatriation. Among these soldiers, there was an alarmingly high rate of appendicitis— about one case every two to three weeks. Even the Japanese medical officers at the camp were surprised by the number of cases, suggesting to Dr. Black that appendicitis was rare among Japanese troops. Dr. Black suspected that the appendicitis was related to the fact that Japanese soldiers were being fed British rations, which had a very low fiber content compared to the traditional Japanese diet.

Similar observations have been made elsewhere. Case in point: When British and Indian troops were stationed in India from 1936 to 1947, appendicitis was four to six times more common in the British soldiers than in the Indian troops, who ate rations that were three times higher in fiber and contained one third the amount of animal protein than the British diet.

Despite the compelling evidence for dietary influences on appendicitis, many medical experts remain skeptical. Cases of appendicitis have actually fallen worldwide since 1950, and improvements in hygiene and better infection control are often cited as possible reasons for the decline.

Even so, in the United States, some 250,000 appendectomies are performed annually. Although there are some valid reasons for the surgery—such as a confirmed case of appendicitis—at least 20 percent of these procedures turn out to be unnecessary. If your surgeon wants to remove your appendix, make sure there is a good reason such as an accurate diagnosis of appendicitis. CT scans and other advanced forms of x-ray technology are helpful in making a precise diagnosis and eliminating unnecessary surgery.

Bottom line: Eating a high-fiber diet is good medicine, whether or not it helps prevent appendicitis. Try to shoot for 25 to 35 grams of fiber daily from a variety of high-fiber foods, and avoid eating refined or processed carbohydrates.

CONSTIPATION

One of the most common complaints heard by doctors is constipation. Medically speaking, constipation is the passage of hard stools fewer than three times a week. Other symptoms such as abdominal bloating and discomfort may accompany constipation, too.

Although constipation is not usually serious, it can incite worrisome complications:

- Intestinal obstruction, which can be a medical emergency.

- Hemorrhoids, a cluster of dilated veins in swollen tissue around the anus.

- Hernia, which occurs when an organ protrudes through the wall of the cavity that normally surrounds it.

- Irritable bowel syndrome, a condition characterized by

alternating periods of diarrhea and constipation, often accompanied by cramping.

- Colon or rectal cancer. With chronic constipation, fecal matter stays in your system too long. The more slowly this material passes through your colon, the higher your colon's exposure to any carcinogens in the waste. This can stimulate abnormal cell growth in your colon and rectum.

What causes constipation, exactly? The major culprit is not eating enough fiber, pure and simple. Other causes include inactivity and poor water intake. Constipation can also be the result of certain diseases, such as kidney failure, colon or rectal cancer, diverticulosis (see below), thyroid problems, prolonged bed rest, and stress. Certain medications cause constipation, including antacids, antihistamines, aspirin, blood pressure medications, diuretics, iron or calcium supplements, and mood-lifting drugs.

Changing your diet to include more fiber-rich foods such as beans, bran, high-fiber cereals, fruits, vegetables, and whole grains should correct constipation and stop it from occurring in the first place. Some of the best foods for increasing regularity are wheat bran, fruits, and vegetables. Other lifestyle changes such as becoming more active and drinking at least eight glasses of pure water a day will also keep you regular.

It is perfectly normal to get constipated every once in a while, but notify your doctor if your constipation continues more than three weeks, even after increasing your fiber intake, water intake, and exercise level. Chronic constipation should always be evaluated by your physician.

DIVERTICULOSIS AND DIVERTICULITIS

Diverticulosis develops when small outpouchings called diverticula, ranging from the size of a piece of confetti to a quarter, form in the colon. Between 20 and 50 percent of all people age 50 and over have diverticulosis. And if you live to age 90, you will have developed some diverticulosis.

Most of the time, it is not a problem. But trouble starts when these diverticula become infected and inflamed, often the result of bacteria, undigested food, or feces becoming lodged within them. The consequences can range from a small abscess to a massive infection or even a perforation of the colon wall. In extreme cases, diverticulitis is life-threatening, should an inflamed diverticulum rupture or perforate and spill intestinal material into the abdominal cavity. This can cause peritonitis, an inflammation of the membrane that covers the abdominal organs. Peritonitis is a medical emergency.

Diverticulosis is generally caused by a low-fiber diet. A diet deficient in fiber produces smaller volumes of stool. To move the smaller stool along the colon and out the rectum, the colon narrows itself by contracting down forcefully. This increases pressure, and over time, high pressure weakens the muscular wall of the colon, causing diverticula to form.

Considering that a majority of people never experience any symptoms, how do you know whether you have diverticulosis? Most diverticulosis is accidentally discovered during routine intestinal tract examinations, such as a barium enema or colonoscopy. Some people with diverticulosis, however, do have symptoms, including constipation, cramping, and bloating. If you have been diagnosed with diverticulosis and suddenly experience pain accompanied by fever, you might be having an attack of diverticulitis. Notify your physician immediately.

Treatment for diverticulitis usually involves hospitalization, in which you receive intravenous antibiotics and a liquid diet to rest your colon. In extreme cases, surgery to remove a section of the colon might be required.

The best way keep diverticulosis from starting, getting worse, or progressing to diverticulitis is by eating a high-fiber diet. Fiber widens the colon, easing the pressure and reducing the chances that existing diverticula will rupture or become inflamed. Two of the best carbs you can eat for preventing or managing diverticulosis are bran cereal and whole-wheat bread.

DUODENAL ULCERS

A duodenal ulcer is a hole or break in the first part of the small intestine known as the duodenum. These ulcers are two to three times more common than those that form in the stomach (gastric ulcer). They develop when there is an imbalance between the amount of natural gastric acid secretions and the resistance to those secretions by the protective intestinal lining in your body. When the normal balance breaks down, the lining is injured, and the result is an ulcer.

A bacteria called *H. pylori* that lives in the mucous membranes lining the digestive tract is the most common cause of duodenal ulcers. About 95 percent of patients with this type of ulcer are infected with *H. pylori*. Also, the regular use of painkillers, mainly nonsteroidal anti-inflammatory drugs (NSAIDs), such as aspirin and ibuprofen, can increase your risk of developing an ulcer by as much as 40 percent. Smoking is another major risk factor.

Symptoms of a duodenal ulcer include heartburn, a burning sensation in the back of the throat, or stomach pain. Bloating and nausea after meals are common complaints, too.

The usual treatment for ulcers is medication to decrease the amount of acid produced or to coat the lining of your duodenum for protection. In addition, many doctors recommend treatment to eliminate *H. pylori*. The usual therapy involves antibiotics and Pepto-Bismol.

But high-fiber nutrition might play a role, too, and is often recommended as a preventive measure. Fiber might promote healing and prevent a recurrence of the ulcer, according to a study conducted at the Harvard School of Public Health. Although the reason for this ulcer-curbing benefit is unclear, researchers speculate that fiber somehow helps keep the duodenal lining intact by balancing the gastric juices and the resistance of that lining to injury.

Another Harvard study found that fiber protects against the formation of duodenal ulcers. In this study, researchers followed 48,000 men over a 6-year period and observed that those who averaged 30 grams of fiber a day cut their risk of duodenal ulcers in half. A higher intake of vitamin A was also linked to fewer ulcers. High-fiber foods such as apricots, peaches, prunes, carrots, and pumpkin are plentiful in vitamin A and, thus, might deliver a one-two punch against duodenal ulcers. The take-home message here is: Eat a high-fiber diet, with plenty of vitamin A-rich foods, to ward off this digestive disease.

GALLSTONES

Situated beneath the liver is a pear-shape organ called the gallbladder. It serves a useful purpose—storing bile, a greenish fluid that contains bile acids and cholesterol. Required for the breakdown and digestion of fats, bile is secreted by the liver and makes its way into the small intestine via a passageway called the bile duct.

If cholesterol in the bile duct gets too high, gallstones can form in the gallbladder. These are crystal-like structures that might be as small as a grain of sand or as large as a golf ball. Most gallstones are practically pure cholesterol. They can migrate to other parts of the digestive tract, causing severe pain and life-threatening complications. In rare cases, severe inflammation can cause the gallbladder to rupture, which can be fatal.

If your doctor suspects you have gallstones, you'll undergo blood tests for liver enzyme levels. These levels are usually elevated with gallbladder disease. A definitive diagnosis is made through ultrasound.

Treatment for gallstones varies, depending upon the severity of the situation. Sometimes gallstones can be dissolved by taking bile acids in tablet form or broken up through high-frequency sound waves in a procedure known as lithotripsy. Where there is a severe obstruction and pain, your surgeon might elect to remove the entire gallbladder in a procedure called a cholecystecomy.

Although the gallbladder serves a useful function, the body can get along without it. Still, any type of surgery is stressful on your body, particularly your immune system. One study found an elevated risk of colon cancer following gallbladder removal. Fortunately though, the risk disappears after fourteen years. But if facing gallbladder surgery, seek a second opinion.

The best course of action against gallstones is to prevent them from ever forming. Studies show that eating a poor diet—one that is high in fat, processed foods, sugar, and meat and low in fiber and good carbohydrates—increases your odds of getting gallstones. So it is best to follow a diet that is high in fiber and low in fats, especially saturated fats. Olive oil is recommended (no more than two tablespoons a day) as a healthy fat to include in your diet; it helps lower cholesterol levels in the blood and in the gallbladder. What's more, try to replace processed foods and other bad carbs with complex carbohydrates such as whole grains.

HEMORRHOIDS

*Anal and rectal blood vessels form a tight seal that pre-*vents stool from leaking out, but when these vessels be-come swollen, often the result of straining during a bowel movement, hemorrhoids form. They can often rupture, causing bleeding.

There are two types of hemorrhoids: those that occur internally near the beginning of the anal canal, and those that occur externally, extending just outside the anus. Once hemorrhoids develop in either of these locations, itching, pain, and bleeding can arise. If you see bright red blood on your toilet paper, in the toilet bowl, or on the stool itself, a visit to your doctor is imperative. The blood could be related to other serious problems, including can-cer of the colon or rectum.

As with so many other digestive disorders, the best treatment is a high-fiber diet. By reducing constipation, fiber decreases the likelihood of further hemorrhoids de-veloping. Other remedies to relieve the discomfort include the use of over-the-counter suppositories or ointments to lubricate the rectum and anus for smoother passage of stools, warm baths to shrink the swollen blood vessels, and regular exercise.

IRRITABLE BOWEL SYNDROME

*Sometimes called "spastic colon," irritable bowel syn-*drome (IBS) is actually a collection of troublesome symp-toms: constipation, diarrhea, gas, painful bloating, and nausea. In some cases, you have urgent diarrhea first thing in the morning or during and after meals. In others, you experience painful constipation, which alternates with di-arrhea. The good news about IBS, though, is that it is not life-threatening. Nor does it mean that you are at risk for more serious digestive problems.

Women with IBS outnumber men three to one, although no one knows why. Chronic stress and depression trigger IBS symptoms, so part of the problem might be in the mind.

But IBS isn't all mental. It's also in the intestines. In IBS, there is an abnormal muscular activity of the intestinal wall, with bowel muscles contracting up to nine times a minute rather than the normal three. This activity stretches the intestinal wall, causing pain.

Although there is no cure for IBS, you can minimize its symptoms through lifestyle changes such as exercise, stress management, and diet. A high-fiber diet will help relieve the constipation and diarrhea; however, you have to select foods carefully. Beans, for example, can cause unpleasant gas. A small amount of the carbs in beans comes from sugars, namely raffinose, stachyose, and verabose. These sugars are the culprits in the intestinal problems associated with beans. The small intestine doesn't have the right enzymes to digest these sugars, so they arrive in the large intestine undigested. Bacteria residing there have a heyday feeding off these sugars and fermenting them. Carbon dioxide, hydrogen, and other gases are given off in the process. You can relieve discomfort caused by undigested sugars by using a product called Beano, an enzyme preparation that does the digesting for you.

Beans aren't the only gas-producing carbs. Others are onions, celery, carrots, raisins, prune juice, and Brussels sprouts. Never suddenly increase the fiber in your diet; start with small doses so your bowel gets used to it.

Your physician might also recommend that you take a bulk former, such as Metamucil, which contains the natural vegetable fiber psyllium. It might also help relieve your constipation and diarrhea.

PREBOTICS: A SPECIAL CARBOHYDRATE FOR DIGESTIVE HEALTH

Fiber is not the only nondigestible remnant found in carbohydrates that makes its way through your system. Others are "prebotics," a special type of undigested carbohydrate that help promote the growth of friendly bacteria in your gut while curtailing colonies of harmful bacteria. Technically, prebiotics are known as "fructooligosaccharides." Yes, that's a mouthful, so they've been nicknamed FOS for short. This carbohydrate is found naturally in many foods, including bananas, tomatoes, Jerusalem artichokes, onions, garlic, and various whole grains. If you eat a variety of these foods, you take in approximately 800 milligrams of FOS a day. So beneficial is this carbohydrate that it is increasingly being added to certain foods, such as juices, to provide a health benefit beyond the traditional nutrients a particular food contains.

After reaching your colon, FOS becomes a "meal" for health-promoting bacteria (known as probiotics), believed to enhance healthy flora in the intestines, improve digestion, and prevent disease. In other words, these good bacteria feed on FOS, and this results in increasing their numbers in the colon. (Bad bacteria, incidentally, do not feed on FOS.)

Increasing your consumption of prebiotics, whether through food or supplements, offers several benefits. Prebiotics:

* Increase good bacteria while reducing bad bacteria.

* Stimulate the absorption of water and minerals.

* Improve digestive health.

* Prevent certain types of diarrhea.

- Protect liver function.

- Reduce cholesterol and high blood pressure.

Supplementing with Prebiotics

Many health experts believe that Americans do not consume enough FOS-containing foods and recommend that we need about three times more than we currently eat. That being so, these important prebiotics are added to certain foods and found in a growing number of dietary supplements.

Prebiotics are available supplementally in capsules and in loose powder form. They are also cropping up in dietary beverages such as Ensure and other liquid carbohydrate supplements. The recommended dosage for pure FOS is 2,000 to 3,000 milligrams a day. Prebiotics are generally safe; the only reported side effect from supplementation is gas and bloating.

PLEASE PASS THE FIBER: PRESCRIPTION FOR PREVENTION

*High-fiber diets maintain the health of your digestive sys-*tem and help it run smoothly. For a diet to earn the title of "high fiber," it must supply between 25 to 35 grams of fiber daily. If you weigh 175 pounds or more, you would want to shoot for even more fiber, say 40 to 45 grams a day. From information in chapter 2, you know there are two types of fiber—soluble and insoluble—and you should try to include both types in your diet by eating a variety of fruits, vegetables, cereals, and whole grains.

Getting 25 to 35 grams, or more, of fiber in your daily diet is not difficult. Start your day with a high-fiber breakfast, and you will be well on your way to meeting your daily fiber objective without really thinking about it or doing bothersome calculations. Try to eat a cereal for breakfast that has at least 4 grams of fiber per serving. Add to that cereal a high-fiber fruit such as raspberries (8 grams per cup) or blueberries (also 8 grams per cup), and you can meet nearly half the recommended fiber intake first thing in the morning. The rest of the day, choose one or two more fruits, several servings of vegetables, a slice or two of high-fiber bread (it should have 3 grams of fiber per slice), and a serving of legumes, and you will automatically serve up a high-fiber day for yourself. The following table identifies several high-fiber cereals that are good choices for breakfast to get your day started right.

HIGH-FIBER JUMP-STARTS

	High-Fiber Breakfast Cereals	Fiber Grams Per Serving
General Mills	Fiber One—½ cup	14
	Multi-Bran Chex—1 cup	6.4
	Total Raisin Bran—1 cup	5
	Oatmeal Crisp with Almonds—1 cup	4
Kellogg's	All Bran with Extra Fiber—½ cup	13
	Fiberwise—½ cup	10
	All Bran—½ cup	9.7
	Bran Chex—1 cup	8
	Whole-Grain Shredded Wheat—¼ cup	8
	Cracklin' Oat Bran—¾ cup	6.5
	Bran Flakes—¾ cup	4.6
Post	100% Bran—⅓ cup	8
	Raisin Bran—1 cup	8
	Shredded Wheat and Bran—1¼ cup	8
	Bran Flakes—¾ cup	5
	Fruit & Fibre—¾ cup	5
	Grape Nuts—½ cup	5
	Shredded Wheat Original—2 biscuits	5

EIGHT

Heart-Healthy Carbs

The old news is that a low-fat diet helps reduce your risk of heart disease. The new news is that a low-sugar diet does, too.

It's true that the mainline dietary strategy for fighting heart trouble centers around cutting out fat-ridden foods. That's essential. But reducing fat alone does not necessarily decrease your risk of heart disease. You have to limit the amount of added, refined sugar you eat, too, and that's what we will be focusing on in this chapter.

For background, heart disease is the nation's leading killer. Nearly 2,600 Americans die of it each day, an average of 1 death every 33 seconds. And if you have diabetes, this can double or quadruple your risk; heart disease is the number-one cause of death among diabetics. Although heart disease might build up over many years, its impact can be quite sudden, often resulting in a heart attack.

The blood vessels that provide oxygen and nutrients to the heart muscle encircle the heart like a crown, which is why they're called "coronary arteries." Problems begin when fatty deposits called plaque build up or a clot lodges in the artery, narrowing the passageway and choking off blood flow. A symptom of plaque buildup is angina, or chest pain. It's usually one of the first warning signs of coronary heart disease. (Other symptoms are listed in the following box.) A heart attack occurs when blood flow to the heart muscle is cut off for a long period of time and part of the heart muscle dies.

CLASSIC SYMPTOMS OF HEART DISEASE

- A squeezing sensation in the chest that feels like a fist clenching your heart.

- A heaviness in the chest

- Pain that radiates from the chest into the neck, shoulders, stomach, or back and doesn't go away

- Shortness of breath

- Intense sweating

- Fainting

With heart disease, prevention is paramount, and one of the many dietary measures you can take is to restrict the amount of sugar in your diet, and replace it with more healthy, wholesome carbohydrates. (Some of the other major preventive steps are listed in the following box.) When I talk about "sugar," I'm referring to added sugar, the stuff that is used to sweeten soft drinks and incorporated into other foods. Added sugar is a bad carb that should be limited in your diet. As I mentioned earlier, the average person eats a half-pound or more of added sugar a day. That's too much if you want to keep your ticker in top condition.

LIVING A HEART-HEALTHY LIFESTYLE

Preventing and managing heart disease involves mostly lifestyle changes, including diet, that can drastically reduce your risk. One is to quit smoking. Smoking is public enemy number one when it comes to heart health. It strains the heart by constricting the arteries and making it beat faster. It elevates blood pressure and increases poisonous carbon monoxide in the blood.

- High blood pressure is a risk factor too. Even with a diagnosis of mild high blood pressure, you triple your risk of heart attack. Many times you don't even know you have high blood pressure until you have it checked.

- If you're overweight, try to trim down. Extra pounds are hard on your heart. The higher your weight climbs, the greater your risk. Being overweight also raises blood pressure and cholesterol, which are risk factors themselves. Even a weight loss of just ten pounds can improve your risk status. Maintaining weight is important, too. Cycling up and down in weight puts you at a greater risk. So does your body shape. If you're built like an apple, with extra pounds around your middle, you're at a greater risk.

- A low-fat diet will help you lose weight, too. Plus, it helps control cholesterol—another major risk factor in heart disease. The higher the level of LDL cholesterol in your blood, the greater your chances that plaque will build up in your arteries. Eating too much saturated fat, like animal fats, butter, and high-fat dairy products, can drive your cholesterol levels way up.

- Talk to your doctor about aspirin therapy. Aspirin reduces inflammation in the body. Plus, it is an "antiplatelet drug," which means it prevents platelets—tiny clotting substances in blood—from abnormally clumping together in a process called platelet aggregation. Platelet aggregation triggers the formation of dangerous blood clots called thrombi (or thrombus in the singular).

SUGAR AND YOUR HEART

The link between the consumption of refined sugar and heart disease was discovered in the 1940s and 1950s, when researchers found that the prevalence of heart disease was highest in countries where people ate the most sugar. Since then, much more has been learned about sugar and its effect on the heart. Sugar is harmful to your heart for at least six reasons.

Reason #1: Sugar Promotes Inflammation

Sugar weakens your body's resistance to bacteria, viruses, and yeasts—all of which cause inflammation in both the heart and arteries. Inflammation plays a role in the build-up of artery-clogging plaque and is now recognized as a major risk factor for heart disease.

Inflammation is a bodily immune response that is triggered when your body is under attack from germs and other invaders. The immune system presses cells into service to destroy the invaders. Inside blood vessels, these cells can pile up, forming lesions that might eventually rupture and lead to a heart attack if preventive measures, mostly involving lifestyle changes, are not undertaken.

You can be tested for inflammation with a simple blood test that measures C-reactive protein (CRP), a protein that increases with the amount of inflammation in your coronary arteries. High levels of CRP are now believed to be the strongest and most significant predictors of heart disease, heart attack, and stroke.

One way to reduce inflammation in your body is to cut back or avoid high-sugar foods, as well as fatty meat, another inflammation-triggering food. A low intake of fruits and vegetables sets the stage for inflammation; so does not exercising. With some simple dietary and lifestyle changes, you can go a long way toward halting inflammation so it does not damage your heart and blood vessels.

Reason #2: Sugar Elevates Triglycerides

Synthesized in the liver, triglycerides are the form in which fat travels through your bloodstream. When there is too much of this fat en route through your system, the excess gradually finds its way to your inner arterial walls, where it is deposited, eventually obstructing your arteries. Two major dietary factors are known to elevate triglycerides: eating too much saturated fat (the type found mainly in animal foods) and eating too much added sugar. Several other factors beside sugar and saturated fat can elevate your triglyceride levels: drinking alcohol, smoking, taking estrogen, and following a diet high in other bad carbs.

When you have your cholesterol checked and analyzed, your triglycerides are checked and measured also. Any number lower than 150 is considered normal for triglycerides; higher numbers are considered a risk factor for heart disease. The following table lists healthy and unhealthy ranges for triglycerides.

TRIGLYCERIDE READINGS

Normal triglycerides	Less than 150
Borderline high triglycerides	150 to 199
High triglycerides	200 to 499
Very high triglycerides	500 or greater

Source: American Heart Association

If you have high triglycerides, you might also have elevated LDL cholesterol, because the two often go hand in hand. LDL cholesterol is a type of fat produced in your liver, usually in response to an excess of saturated fat in your diet. Essentially, too much saturated fat disrupts your liver's ability to break down cholesterol, so it churns out LDL cholesterol, which can form lesions inside your arteries. LDL cholesterol is considered the "bad" cholesterol. You might also have too-low levels of HDL cholesterol (considered the good kind). When triglyceride levels are too high, HDL cholesterol tends to fall.

How exactly does sugar increase triglyceride levels? The more sugar you eat, the higher and faster it increases glucose in your blood. This causes your pancreas to pump out more insulin to lower your blood sugar. Insulin is fat-promoting hormone. Secreting a lot of it prevents your body from burning fat, including triglycerides, and consequently, your liver converts the glucose into triglycerides and releases them into your bloodstream. Sugar isn't the only food to trigger this reaction. Eating a lot of carbohydrates that are high on the glycemic index—in other words, foods that quickly raise blood sugar—also causes increased production of triglycerides.

As I explained in chapter 2, one of the most damaging types of added sugar is fructose, mainly in the form of high-fructose corn syrup, a refined version of fructose made from corn and found in many processed foods and so-called health foods. Fructose is fat-forming in the body because it is metabolized differently than other sugars are.

Reducing your triglycerides requires revamping your lifestyle to reduce the amount of sugar you eat (including high-fructose corn syrup), cut back on the saturated fat in your diet, avoid or limit alcohol consumption, and become more active. For your fat source, consider substituting monounsaturated fats such as olive oil or canola oil. In research, both have been shown to lower triglyceride levels.

Reason #3: Sugar Affects Concentrations of Protective HDL Cholesterol

A heart-friendly cholesterol is high-density lipoprotein, or HDL cholesterol. Its job is to pick up the bad cholesterol from the cells in the artery walls and transport it back to the liver for reprocessing or excretion from the body as waste. HDL cholesterol has been nicknamed the "good cholesterol."

Eating "slow" carbohydrates—those low on the glycemic index—might positively affect concentrations of this good cholesterol—so says a British study of the dietary habits of 1,420 men and women. The researchers discovered that those who had diets rich in low-glycemic index foods, such as beans, had higher levels of HDL cholesterol.

By contrast, diets consisting of higher-glycemic index carbs drive HDL levels down. The reason for this has to do with insulin. Continually choosing sugar and quick-digesting carbs or large amounts of these foods—which are high on the glycemic index—raises blood sugar and insulin levels. High insulin contributes to low HDL cholesterol levels.

If your cholesterol profile is out of whack—that is, too-low HDL levels and too-high LDL levels—you might try eating low-glycemic index carbs for a few months to see if this makes any difference. Support this dietary change with other lifestyle measures, such as following a diet low in saturated fat and getting regular exercise.

Reason #4: Sugar Influences Obesity

Having a weight problem raises your blood sugar, your cholesterol, and your blood pressure, all of which are major risk factors for heart disease.

If you want to get your weight under control and avoid

the health problems related to being overweight and
obese, you must definitely restrict your sugar intake.
When eaten in excess, sugar has a tendency to be converted into body fat. Sugar is rapidly released into your
system, driving your blood sugar up too high and giving
you a quick "rush," followed by a fast "crash." The first
organ to react to this sugar overload is the pancreas, which
responds by secreting more insulin into your bloodstream.
Insulin activates fat cell enzymes, facilitating the movement of fat from the bloodstream into fat cells for storage.
Additionally, insulin prevents glucagon (a hormone that
opposes the action of insulin) from entering the bloodstream, and glucagon is responsible for unlocking fat
stores. The cumulative result of these interactions is the
ready conversion of simple sugars to body fat. If you need
to lose weight, see chapter 9 for an effective way to trim
down and still enjoy carbohydrates.

Reason #5: Sugar Robs Your Body of Important B Vitamins

Vital for energy, B vitamins are involved in nearly every
reaction in the body, from the manufacture of new red
blood cells to the metabolism of carbohydrates, fat, and
protein. In excess, sugar leads to deficiencies in all the B
vitamins, which are essential for healthy arteries.

Certain B vitamins—namely folate, vitamin B_6, and vitamin B_{12}—are needed to prevent the buildup of homocysteine in the blood. Homocysteine is a harmful
substance that causes the cells lining arterial walls to deteriorate, leading to heart attack or stroke. A deficiency
of vitamin B_6, in particular, leads to atherosclerosis.

Another important heart-helper is the B vitamin niacin.
It is involved in the regulation of cholesterol and triglyceride levels.

With the exception of vitamin B_{12} (found mostly in

protein foods), whole grains and vegetables are rich sources of B vitamins. Make sure your diet serves up plenty of these foods to protect yourself against deficiencies.

Reason #6: Sugar Promotes the Formation of AGEs

When your body is subjected to high levels of glucose—which can happen if you're eating a lot of sugar as a matter of habit—sugar rushing into the bloodstream as glucose links up (or glycates) with proteins in the body. The by-products of this reaction are the compounds called advanced glycation end products (AGEs), which can inflict damage in your body. AGEs alter tissue proteins, weakening bodily tissue (including blood vessels), reducing the elasticity of tissues, and interfering with normal cellular functions. All these situations can conspire to increase your risk of heart disease.

LDL cholesterol can become glycated, too—a process that prevents the normal shutdown of cholesterol synthesis in the liver. As a result, cholesterol levels soar, increasing the risk of atherosclerosis (the narrowing and thickening of arteries). Also, AGEs generate health-damaging free radicals.

The bottom line: When blood glucose is chronically elevated, there is a glut of glycated cells and substances in your system. Your body can't handle the excess, and the risk of health problems, including heart disease, is bound to increase. Slash the sugar to slash your risk.

KIND-HEARTED STRATEGIES

Clearly, a poor diet is a major cause of heart trouble, but you can do something about it. To improve your heart health and reduce your risk of heart disease, keep an eye

on the kind of carbohydrates you eat, along with watching
your fat intake. For best protection:

• Reduce the amount of sugar you eat by avoiding bad
  carbs such as soft drinks, candy, pastry, and high-sugar
  cereals. Limit desserts to twice a week and try to stick
  to lower-fat desserts. Have fresh fruit for dessert more
  often. Drink unsweetened beverages. If you have a
  sweet tooth, use artificial sweeteners instead of caving
  in to your sugar urge. There's a new one on the market
  called Tagatose, and it is discussed at the end of this
  chapter.

• Limit your intake of fat-free commercial foods. These
  might be low in fat, but they are often loaded with
  added sugar and calories.

• If your triglycerides are high or your HDL cholesterol
  is too low, try eating carbs that are low on the glycemic
  index (rated 55 or less): barley, high-fiber cereals,
  whole-grain pasta, oat bran, oatmeal, apples, pears, oranges, beans, peas, and sweet potatoes. These carbs are
  absorbed more slowly into the bloodstream. Slower absorption restrains surges in insulin release and slows
  the production of triglycerides in the liver. Stay on a
  diet like this for a few months; then have your blood
  fats (triglycerides and cholesterol) tested to see if this
  dietary strategy works for you.

• Follow a high-fiber diet. Studies show that people who
  eat the most dietary fiber (in carbs such as high-fiber
  cereals, whole grains, fruits, and vegetables) have the
  lowest death rates due to heart disease. Although a
  high-fiber diet means between 25 and 35 grams of fiber
  a day, you can protect your heart with as few as 16
  grams a day. That's the finding of one major study in

which people who ate 16 grams of fiber daily had one-third the risk of dying of heart disease as those who ate less than 16 grams. The reason fiber works so powerfully is threefold. Soluble fiber (in foods such as oat bran, beans, and apples) is very effective at lowering cholesterol. Plus, fiber is believed to interfere with the formation of blood clots that can trigger heart attack and stroke. This type of fiber also keeps blood glucose in safe bounds. Just a half-cup to a full cup of beans daily can significantly cut your cholesterol and control your blood sugar.

- Improve the quality of carbohydrates you eat by shifting your diet to more good carbs and fewer bad carbs. In the following table, you'll find a list of carbohydrates that are healthiest for your heart. Eat a variety of these foods through the week.

- Balance the amount of carbohydrates you eat with other nutrients. The American Heart Association recommends the following nutrient balance: 55 percent of total calories from carbohydrates, 30 percent or less from fat, and 15 percent from protein.

- Consider going meatless (vegetarian) several times a week. Many studies have proved that a low-fat vegetarian diet not only prevents heart disease, but also can reverse it. In one study, a vegetarian low-fat diet, in which total fat was reduced to 10 percent of calories, along with daily exercise and a stress management program, had dramatic effects on the heart health of patients. After a year, 18 of the 22 patients in the study showed significant clearing in their arteries, plus a 91 percent reduction in the frequency of chest pains. In effect, they had reversed their heart disease.

HEART-PROTECTIVE GOOD CARBS

Good Carbs	How They Work
Barley	Contains soluble fiber, which reduces the absorption of cholesterol, decreases its production in the liver, and increases its elimination in the stool.
Beans and legumes	Rich in soluble fiber, which reduces the absorption of cholesterol, decreases its production in the liver, and increases its elimination in the stool.
Broccoli	Contains vitamin C, which helps keep arteries elastic and blood from clotting abnormally; also high in glutathione, an antioxidant that reduces heart disease risk, plus lowers blood pressure.
Carrots, pumpkin, sweet potatoes, yams, and other orange vegetables	Rich in carotenoids, including beta-carotene. Carotenoids might halt damage to the lining of the arteries.
Citrus fruits and other vitamin C–rich foods	Rich in vitamin C, which helps maintain the integrity of both the blood vessels and the heart muscle.
Fruits and vegetables	May lower levels of C-reactive protein (CRP) in the body, a marker of how inflamed heart arteries might be. High levels of CRP are a strong predictor of heart disease and are associated with blood clots. Fruits and vegetables contain natural antioxidants that might stop the formation of AGEs.
Garlic	May prevent the oxidation of cholesterol—a free-radical-generated process in which fatty streaks form on the inside of artery walls, leading to narrowing of arteries.

(continued)

HEART-PROTECTIVE GOOD CARBS

Good Carbs	How They Work
Green leafy vegetables	High in folate (folic acid), which lowers levels of homocysteine, a substance in the blood that increases the risk of heart disease.
Magnesium-rich carbs (tofu, beans and legumes, whole grains, and green leafy vegetables)	Magnesium is vital for heart health. It helps prevent heart attack, angina, irregular heart beats, high blood pressure, low HDL cholesterol levels, strokes, and overall heart function.
Oats and oat bran	Contain soluble fiber, which reduces the absorption of cholesterol, decreases its production in the liver, and increases its elimination in the stool.
Onions	May prevent the oxidation of cholesterol—a free-radical-generated process in which fatty streaks form on the inside of artery walls, leading to narrowing of arteries.
Soy foods	Lower levels of harmful cholesterol. (Twenty-five grams of soy protein a day is recommended.) Tofu, or soybean curd, has been shown to lower cholesterol in more than thirty-seven studies.
Whole grains	High in vitamin B_6 (pyroxidine), which helps prevent atherosclerosis by lowering homocysteine in the body, preventing abnormal blood clotting, preserving elasticity of blood vessels, normalizing cholesterol levels, and lowering blood pressure.
Whole wheat (including bread)	Helps reduce levels of homocysteine and LDL cholesterol.

Most people find it easier to phase into a vegetarian diet by becoming a partial vegetarian. You can accomplish this with a gradual reduction in the amount of meat you eat. For example, plan several meatless days each week or a meatless meal each day. Another strategy is to become a semi-vegetarian (one who eats dairy foods, eggs, poultry, and fish but no red meat) or a pesco-vegetarian (one who eats dairy foods, eggs, and fish but no other animal flesh) before moving on to the stricter forms of vegetarianism.

To help you make the switch, here are some additional pointers:

- For starters, eliminate red meat but continue to eat poultry and fish occasionally.

- Make complex carbohydrates the centerpiece of your meals, rather than an animal protein.

- Early on, incorporate one vegetarian meal a day into your menus, eventually phasing out flesh foods and making all meals vegetarian.

- Find vegetarian recipes you enjoy.

- Consider "substitute meats"—products made from soybeans that are formed to look and taste like hot dogs, sausage, ground beef, and bacon.

- For variety and good health, include many different foods in your diet, because no single food contains all the nutrients you need.

You should now have a better idea that heart disease is a very real threat but that you can do something about it before it's too late. Cut back on your intake of sugar and saturated fat, eat the right types of carbs, exercise, make other changes in your lifestyle, get regular check-ups, and recognize the symptoms of heart disease. By taking these positive actions, you can live better, and quite possibly, a lot longer.

TAGATOSE

If you're cutting back on sugar yet hate the aftertaste and limitations of artificial sweeteners, you're in for a treat in the form of tagatose, a low-calorie natural sugar that has been recently approved by the FDA for use in foods, beverages, and other products.

Manufactured from lactose, a simple sugar found in milk, tagatose looks like sugar, tastes like sugar, and best of all, cooks like sugar. The major difference between tagatose and sugar is that tagatose has fewer calories (roughly 6 calories per teaspoon compared to 16 calories for sugar) and has a low glycemic response, meaning that it won't push blood sugar and insulin up to unhealthy levels. For that reason, tagatose will probably be widely used as a sweetener in foods formulated for people with diabetes.

In addition, this new sweetener has applications in weight control. In one study, diabetic and normal patients using the sweetener on a daily basis lost weight at a consistent but gradual rate. What's more, tagatose has been shown in research to be a prebiotic, promoting healthy bacteria in the intestines for better digestion. It does not cause cavities either, and might even reduce the risk of tooth decay.

Tagatose is expected to be added to a wide range of foods, including soft drinks, cereals, baked goods, ice cream, candy, and chewing gum. It will also be used in toothpastes, cough syrups, medicines, and cosmetics.

Studied for more than ten years, tagatose appears to have no side effects.

NINE

Carbs and Weight Control:
The Good-Carb Diet

To eat carbs or not to eat carbs.

That is the question on everyone's mind—everyone who wants to lose weight and stay trim, that is. Nowhere have carbohydrates been more bashed as they have been in the arena of weight control. When it comes to overweight and obesity, carbs are the nutritional equivalent of *persona non grata*. Do they deserve such a bad rap? Read on; the answer to that question might surprise you.

CARBOHYDRATES AND OBESITY

*More than two-thirds of the U.S. population is now con-*sidered overweight or obese (weighing 20 percent or more than what is considered a healthy weight), and obesity has become a global epidemic. One of the major nutritional reasons for such widespread (excuse the pun) obesity in America is hiding on the carbohydrate side of the dietary equation. Since low-fat dieting hit the diet scene in the early 1980s, everybody started cutting the fat from their diets while increasing calories from carbohydrates. The diet mantra at the time was: Slash fat, eat carbs. We bought into the low-fat, high-carbohydrate message as hapless participants, but little did we know that we were setting ourselves up for big problems down the road.

Over time, some alarming blips appeared on the nutritional radar screen: People started getting fatter, not thinner. After the government's Food Guide Pyramid (a meal planning guide) was introduced in 1991, sermonizing the value of eating six to eleven servings of carbohydrates a day (including some bad carbs) while eating fats "sparingly," the number of overweight, out-of-shape Americans jumped a whopping 61 percent. We cut the fat from our diets but got wider bottoms and bigger bellies in the process.

Whoa, hold it right there—aren't you supposed to slash fat to lose weight? Isn't low-fat dieting the ticket to a slender life? Isn't it? Not necessarily, say nutritional scientists who have studied the relationship between the simultaneous rise in obesity and the rise in carbohydrate intake.

What appears to be largely responsible for the escalating obesity in our country is that we are eating an excess of bad carbs—foods such as white bread, baked goods, foods with added sugar, and other processed junk foods. The carbohydrate-to-fat ratio in the typical American diet has gotten way out of whack. Bottom line: Eating too much of the wrong kinds of carbs—the bad carbs—can make you fat.

THE PROS AND CONS OF
LOW-CARBOHYDRATE DIETING

Another prevailing reason for carbs' bad rap is that dieters everywhere have gone high-protein, low-carb bon-

kers. I'm willing to wager that there are millions of people right now who are following a high-protein/low-carb diet—and you might be one of the converts. Perhaps even your doctor recommended it. If so, that's bad advice and bad medicine, especially if you care about your health.

I realize that these diets are popular because they let you load up on steak, cheese, and other high-fat fare. But they prohibit many other health-protective foods; most of them are the good carbs I have been encouraging in this book. You know the spiel of these diets: few fruits and vegetables, few carbohydrates.

What's wrong with this type of diet? To begin with, it is very high in fat. Roughly 50 percent or more of its calories come from fat—a lot of it saturated (that's one of the worst of the bad fats). If you are worried about cancer (particularly colon cancer or prostate cancer) or heart disease, you would want to avoid eating this way, because high-fat diets have been linked to numerous cancers and cardiovascular problems.

Also, a diet like this might not supply enough of the calcium you need for good bone health. Calcium is practically flushed out of your body with a high-protein diet.

What's more, the fiber on this type of diet would be miniscule. Eating a low-fiber diet is harmful to your digestive health and is a real invitation to diverticulosis, kidney stones, and gallstones. You'll be popping lots of laxatives, for sure, while on such a diet. Other health-preventive nutrients, such as antioxidants and phytochemicals that are found mostly in fruits and vegetables, would be missing from this diet as well.

There are other penalties, too. On a low-carb diet, your body is deprived of its favorite fuel. You're low on gas and feel it, physically and mentally. In this de-energized state, accompanied by a gloomy mood, it becomes tough to stick to your eating program, and another attempt to lose weight could bite the dust.

Why Low-Carb Dieting Works

When you think about the number of nutrients that aren't being delivered and the health risks involved, you have to ask yourself why in the world would anyone follow such a diet?

The reason you and many other people diet like this is because *low-carbohydrate dieting works*. When you reduce your intake of carbohydrates, your body starts drawing on its fat reserves for energy. Although your body prefers to fuel itself with carbohydrates, it will use fat as a backup if need be.

If you consider that a good deal of obesity is a result of eating too many calories from bad carbs, cutting carbs to lose weight just makes sense. But there's more to it: When you overindulge on bad carbs, your body overproduces insulin in an effort to transport glucose into cells. Medically known as "hyperinsulinemia," high concentrations of insulin trigger your body to create more fat cells. Another problem brought on by a diet high in bad carbs is "insulin resistance," in which insulin can't do its job of processing sugar and fats for energy. Consequently, your body starts storing more fat than is normal.

So by eating fewer carbs, you keep your blood sugar levels low, and insulin functions as it should—no hyperinsulinemia, no insulin resistance. Metabolically, your body is able to tap into its fat stores for energy, your weight starts decreasing, and before long, you're lean as a hairpin. So you see: Low-carb dieting is a very efficient way to shed pounds.

Still, many people are asking this important question: *Isn't there some way I can lose weight fast and effectively and still eat some carbs?* Or asked another way: *Can't I have my carbs and eat them, too?*

Answer: yes!

You can have your carbs and eat them, too, if the carbs

you select are good carbs—and you eat them in the right proportions. You see, where low-carb dieting goes astray is that it advocates cutting too many carbs—even good carbs! The real key to success with low-carb dieting is cutting out bad carbs and reducing fast carbs (high-glycemic carbs), but replacing them with good carbs you love and that won't count against you when it comes to shedding fat.

THE GOOD-CARB DIET

What I'm advocating is a low-bad-carb diet, rather than an out-and-out low-carb diet. This approach is called the Good-Carb Diet, and it combines the principles of low-carb dieting with the principles of good-carb nutrition. When you follow this approach to eating, don't be surprised if you get your cholesterol and your triglycerides under control along with your weight, because shunning bad carbs helps normalize blood fat. Plus, with this method of weight control, you can lose weight effectively, without sacrificing vital nutrients, and energize yourself with a variety of wholesome, healthy carbs.

The Good-Carb Diet takes a five-part fat attack strategy.

1. Eat 120 to 150 Grams of Good Carbs a Day, Including Glycemically Acceptable Carbohydrates

Generally, your body requires roughly 200 grams of carbohydrates a day for peak metabolic functioning. But you can get by with a slight reduction in carbs and still lose weight effectively. The amount of carbohydrates you can eat each day—and encourage your body's fat-burning processes—is approximately 120 to 150 grams a day, or about 480 to 600 calories of good carbohydrates daily. In other words, you do not have to slash your carbohydrate intake to ridiculously low levels like 20 to 50 grams a day in order to drop pounds. You can do it with a healthy, nonsacrificial intake of 120 to 150 grams. That should be welcome news to you if you've been suffering under a very low-carb intake of 50 grams or less!

Among your best choices for weight control are natural, unprocessed carbohydrates ranked 55 or below on the glycemic index of foods. These foods take longer to break down and, consequently, your blood glucose and insulin levels stay relatively constant during the digestion process. This helps control your appetite and boosts fat-burning. High-GI foods, on the other hand, do the opposite. They trigger an insulin spike, causing your body to create more fat cells. High-GI foods also stimulate your appetite. You feel hungry so you're apt to eat more—and more of the wrong foods stimulating your appetite.

Choosing low-GI carbohydrates makes it possible to lose weight more easily. If you base your carbohydrate selections *mostly* on this nutritional element, you will lose weight more quickly than with the same caloric total of other carbohydrates. Refer to chapter 2 for a list of low-GI carbs, and consult the food lists in the following "Good Carbs and Weight Loss" section. Not every carb you eat on the Good-Carb Diet has to necessarily be a low-GI one; simply base a majority of your choices on these foods. Other carbs to choose are what I call "low-starch carbs": salad vegetables, broccoli, cauliflower, green beans, spinach, and so forth. These foods are low in calories and starch and are loaded with health-bestowing nutrients.

2. Increase Your Daily Intake of Fiber

There is an incredibly easy, no-willpower way to manage your weight with good carbs, one that most of us should be doing but aren't: Eat more fiber. More fiber in your diet will help transform your dieting efforts into something so simple and automatic. You'll be able to keep your weight under control without even working at it or making yourself crazy.

For review, fiber (also called "roughage") is the digestion-resistant portion of plant foods. Over the past thirty years, "epidemiologic" studies, in which investigators study large populations of people to see who gets disease and who doesn't, have found that diets low in fiber are linked to a higher risk of obesity. Dietary fiber has several main talents when it comes to weight control:

- **Fiber fills you up but not out.** Soluble fiber, in particular, slows the passage of food from the stomach to the small intestine. This tends to make you feel full after eating. One of the best high-fiber fill-up foods you can eat is oatmeal. Bran and other high-fiber cereals aren't bad, either. In a study conducted at the Veteran's Administration Center in Minneapolis, people who feasted on high-fiber cereal for breakfast ate 150 to 200 less calories at lunch compared to those who had low-fiber breakfasts.

  Another high-fiber heavyweight is the soluble fiber pectin, plentiful in apples, oranges, and bananas. Pectin inflates after soaking up water in the stomach, making you feel full.

- **Fiber promotes satiety.** It takes longer to crunch down on and chew up fibrous foods, so your meals last longer. That's a plus, because it takes about twenty minutes after starting a meal for your body to send signals that it's full. With enough fiber at mealtime, you're less likely to stuff yourself and eat too many calories. What's more, fibrous foods add very few calories to your meals.

* **Fiber stimulates the release of an appetite-suppressing hormone.** The hormone in question is called cholecystokinin (CCK). Secreted by the upper intestines after you eat a meal, CCK acts on nerves in your stomach and slows the rate of digestion. CCK is also released by the hypothalamus, the body's appetite control center. The net effect of CCK's release in your body is to tell your brain you're full. As a result, you feel full during your meal, so again you're less tempted to overeat.

* **Fiber controls your fat and sugar intake.** Fiber-rich diets tend to be low in fat-forming foods such as fats and sugar. By filling up on wholesome, fibrous foods, you have less room for foods that contribute to fat gain.

* **Fiber has a fat-binding effect.** Although fiber slows down the digestion of protein and carbohydrates, it does not do the same with fat. In the digestive system, fibers naturally bind to fats you eat and help escort them from the body, leaving fewer calories left to be stored as body fat.

* **Fiber helps regulate blood sugar.** High-fiber foods require prolonged breakdown and, thus, release blood sugar more slowly. This action helps prevent dips in blood sugar—dips that can lead to food cravings. A high-fiber diet helps maintain even energy levels throughout the day.

* **Fiber produces an automatic caloric deficit.** If you take in 35 grams of fiber a day (recommended for weight loss), you can count on expending nearly 250 calories from the total calories you ate that day. Because fiber makes your body work hard to process it, this actually creates a caloric deficit. You're burning extra calories, but without any extra effort.

• **Fiber increases transit time through your digestive system.** Transit time refers to how fast food moves from entry to exit over the course of digestion and absorption. Fiber in your diet speeds things along, meaning fewer calories are left to be stored as fat.

Fortunately, the carbohydrates you'll be selecting are loaded with this wonder nutrient fiber. The recommended dietary intake for fiber is between 25 and 35 grams a day. Bumping up your intake to the higher end of that range (35 grams) is recommended for weight loss. But do this gradually. If you start eating 35 grams of fiber tomorrow, you will feel bloat, gas, and other intestinal discomfort. Also, drink eight to ten (8 ounces) glasses of plain water every day while following a high-fiber diet. Fiber requires water for proper digestion and elimination.

If you have trouble increasing your fiber, adding a fiber supplement such as Metamucil is an easy way to obtain an additional 6 grams of fiber a day. However, fiber supplements should never replace high-fiber foods. It is always preferable to increase your fiber naturally through good-carb, fiber-rich foods.

3. Balance Your Ratio of Carbohydrates with Other Nutrients in Fat-Burning Proportions

The ratio of carbohydrates, proteins, and fat you eat on a daily basis is very important to effective weight control. A fair body of research indicates that you can lose weight most efficiently when your nutrients are proportioned in approximately the following manner:

• *Carbohydrates:* 40 percent of total daily calories.

• *Protein:* 30 percent of total daily calories

• *Fat:* 30 percent or less of total daily calories.

In a typical 1,200-calorie weight-loss plan, this method of losing fat breaks down in the following manner:

1,200-Calorie Daily Good-Carb Plan

Good carbohydrates: 480 calories from carbohydrates/120 grams of carbohydrates daily. (You can go as high as 150 grams, however, and still lose weight at a steady rate.)

Lean proteins: 360 calories from protein/90 grams of protein daily

Healthy fat: 360 calories from fat/40 (or less) grams of fat daily

4. Modify Your Calories

Although it seems out of "dieting vogue," cutting calories still works wonders for shedding pounds. To lose 1 pound a week (the maximum safe rate of weight loss), you'll need to eat 500 fewer calories a week. If you add calorie-burning exercise to this equation, your weight loss will be even greater. Most people can lose weight safely on a diet that provides 1,200 to 1,500 calories a day.

5. Restrict Starchy Carbohydrates After Your Mid-Day Meal

There is an easy way to trick your body in thinking it is on a low-carb diet—and burn fat in the process: Cut back on certain types of carbs (those with higher-starch content) in the late afternoon and evening. This helps shift your body into a fat-burning mode.

Carbohydrates should be plentiful at breakfast, mid-morning snack time, and lunch meals to provide adequate fuel for the day's activities. But limit carbs at night, when they are less likely to be fully burned from exercise or activity.

GOOD CARBS AND WEIGHT LOSS

Use the following foods to build your meals and lose weight.

The Foods

Low-Glycemic Starches (2 servings daily)

Cereals and Grains

All-Bran cereal

All-Bran with Extra Fiber

Bulgur wheat

Long-grain rice

Oat bran

Old-fashioned oatmeal

Parboiled rice

Pearled barley

Pumpernickel bread

Stone-ground whole-wheat bread

Special K cereal

Whole-grain pasta

Whole-wheat crackers

Beans and Legumes

Black beans

Chickpeas

Kidney beans

Lentils

Lentil soup

Lima beans

Pinto beans

Soybeans

Split peas

Vegetables

Peas

Sweet potatoes

Yams

One serving = ½ cup cooked cereal, rice, or pasta (with ready-to-eat cereals such as Special K, a serving often counts as 1 cup, so read the labels to determine the appropriate serving); 1 slice bread, 1 medium sweet potato or ½ cup mashed sweet potato; ½ cup legumes or peas; or 4 high-fiber, low-fat crackers.

Low-Starch Vegetables (3 to 5 servings daily)

Alfalfa sprouts

All salad vegetables

Arugula

Asparagus

Bamboo shoots

Bok choy

Broccoli

Brussels sprouts

Cabbage

Cauliflower

Celery

Collard greens

Cucumber

Eggplant

Endive

Green beans

Jalapeño or other hot pepper

Leeks

Lettuce, all varieties

Mushrooms

Parsley

Pepper, sweet

Radishes

Scallions

Spinach

Summer squash

Swiss chard

Tomato

Tomato juice

Turnip greens

Water chestnuts

Wax beans

One serving = 1 cup raw vegetables, ½ cup cooked vegetables, or 1 cup vegetable juice.

Glycemically Acceptable Fruits (2 to 3 servings daily)

Apples

Bananas

Blackberries

Blueberries

Cherries

Dried apricots

Grapefruit

Grapes

Kiwifruit

Melons

Oranges

Peaches

Pears

Plums

Prunes

Raspberries

Strawberries

Tangerines

Tangelos

One serving = 1 medium apple, banana, or orange; ½ cup berries; ½ grapefruit; ½ cup frozen or canned (in juice or water) unsweetened fruit; or ¼ cup dried fruit.

Lean Protein (2 servings)

Chicken (skin removed)

Eggs or egg whites

Fish

Lean cuts of beef

Reduced-fat lunch meats

Shellfish

Tofu

Turkey (skin removed)

One serving = 3 to 4 ounces chicken, turkey, fish, shellfish, or lean beef; 2 slices reduced-fat lunch meat; 1 egg; 4 egg whites; or 2 ounces tofu.

Light Dairy Foods (2 servings)

Cottage or ricotta cheese, low-fat

Low-fat milk

Low-fat yogurt

Nonfat yogurt

Skim milk

Soy milk

Reduced-fat cheeses

One serving = 1 cup skim milk, low-fat milk, or soy milk; 1 cup low-fat or nonfat yogurt; ¼ cup cottage or ricotta cheeses; or 2 ounces reduced-fat cheeses.

Healthy Fats (1 serving)

Butter

Margarine (choose "trans-free" products)

Mayonnaise

Reduced-fat margarine or mayonnaise

Reduced-fat or low-calorie salad dressing

Salad dressing

Unoiled nuts and seeds

Vegetable oil (olive or canola oils are best)

One fat serving = 1 tablespoon margarine, butter, mayonnaise, or vegetable oil; 1 tablespoon salad dressing; 2 tablespoons reduced-fat or low-calorie salad dressing, margarine, or mayonnaise; 1 tablespoon unoiled, unsalted nuts and seeds. (You may use nonfat salad dressings more liberally—3 to 4 tablespoons per day, if you wish.)

Using the above food lists, here is a "template" to help you plan your daily menu:

Breakfast

1 serving of a high-fiber cereal

1 serving light dairy

1 serving of a lean protein (optional for breakfast)

1 serving fruit

Snack

1 serving light dairy

1 serving fruit

Lunch

1 serving lean protein

1 serving low-starch carbohydrate

1 serving low-glycemic carbohydrate

1 serving healthy fat

Dinner

1 serving lean protein

1–2 servings low-starch carbohydrate

Sample Seven-Day Plan

Monday

Breakfast

½ cup cooked oatmeal

4 scrambled egg whites

1 cup skim milk

½ grapefruit

Snack

1 cup nonfat yogurt mixed with 1 cup blueberries and
1 tablespoon low-calorie fruit preserves

Lunch
Tuna salad made with 4 ounces water-packed tuna, 1
cup lettuce, 1 tomato slice, and 2 tablespoons low-
calorie Italian salad dressing

1 cup nonfat vegetable soup

½ cup long-grained rice

Dinner
4 ounces roasted chicken breast, skin removed

1 cup asparagus

1 cup spinach

Nutritional information: 1,100 calories; 120 grams carbohydrate; 112 grams protein; 23 grams fat; and 20
grams fiber.

Tuesday

Breakfast
½ cup cooked oat bran

1 cup skim milk

1 banana

Snack
1 cup nonfat yogurt mixed with 1 cup strawberries

Lunch
Spinach salad made with 2 ounces reduced-fat feta
cheese, 1 cup chopped raw spinach, assorted raw
chopped salad vegetables, ½ cup garbanzo beans, and
2 tablespoons low-calorie French dressing

Dinner
4 ounces roasted turkey breast, skin removed

1 cup broccoli, cooked

1 cup summer squash, cooked

Nutritional information: 1,100 calories; 145 grams carbohydrate; 78 grams protein; 35 grams fat; and 31 grams fiber.

Wednesday

Breakfast
1 slice high-fiber toast

1 egg, poached

1 cup low-fat milk

1 orange, medium

Snack
1 cup nonfat yogurt

1 cup sliced fresh raspberries

Lunch
4 ounces roasted chicken breast, skin removed

1 tossed salad

Salad dressing prepared with 1 tablespoon vegetable oil and 2 tablespoons vinegar

½ cup mashed sweet potatoes

1 kiwifruit

Dinner
4 ounces baked cod

1 cup cauliflower, cooked

1 cup yellow wax beans, cooked

Nutritional information: 1,200 calories; 121 grams carbohydrate; 90 grams protein; 33 grams fat; and 25 grams fiber.

Thursday

Breakfast
½ cup All-Bran with Extra Fiber

1 cup soy milk

1 orange, medium

Snack
Smoothie, blended with 1 cup low-fat milk and 1 cup frozen blueberries

Lunch
Open-faced sandwich, prepared with 2 slices reduced-fat turkey ham, sliced tomato, lettuce leaf, 1 tablespoon brown mustard, and 1 slice high-fiber bread

1 cup nonfat vegetable soup

½ cup sliced peaches, water-packed

Dinner
5 ounces grilled salmon

1 tossed salad with 2 tablespoons low-calorie French dressing

1 cup turnip greens, cooked

Nutritional information: 1,100 calories; 134 grams carbohydrate; 72 grams protein; 34 grams fat; and 39 grams fiber.

Friday

Breakfast
1 cup Special K

1 cup low-fat milk

1 cup fresh raspberries

Snack
4 whole-wheat crackers, spread with ¼ cup low-fat cottage cheese

Lunch
Chicken Caesar salad, prepared with 3 ounces chicken breast, 1 cup chopped romaine lettuce, 1 sliced small green pepper, 3 tablespoons chopped onion, and 1 tablespoon Caesar salad dressing

½ cup fruit cocktail, water-packed

Dinner
4 ounces grilled rib eye steak

1 cup mixed vegetables

1 cup stewed tomatoes

Nutritional information: 1,232 calories; 144 grams carbohydrate; 83 grams protein; 40 grams fat; and 30 grams fiber.

Saturday

Breakfast
One egg, scrambled

1 slice high-fiber toast

1 cup low-fat milk

½ grapefruit

Snack
1 cup nonfat yogurt

1 apple, medium

Lunch
Chili prepared with ½ cup kidney beans, 3 ounces lean ground beef, and 1 cup cooked tomatoes with green chilies

1 tossed salad with 1 tablespoon low-fat salad dressing

1 cup melon balls

Dinner
5 ounces steamed shrimp

½ cup coleslaw prepared with 1 tablespoon low-fat slaw dressing

1 cup broccoli

Nutritional information: 1,200 calories; 129 grams carbohydrate; 100 grams protein; 35 grams fat; and 23 grams fiber.

Sunday

Breakfast
½ cup All-Bran with Extra Fiber

1 cup nonfat yogurt

1 cup fresh raspberries

Snack
Soy smoothie blended with 1 cup soy milk and ½ cup frozen peaches

Lunch
Chicken chef salad prepared with 4 ounces baked chicken, 1 cup chopped lettuce, 1 cup chopped assorted salad vegetables, and 2 tablespoons low-calorie French dressing

1 slice high-fiber bread

Dinner
4 ounces baked turkey breast, no skin

1 cup cooked summer squash

1 cup cooked broccoli

Nutritional information: 1,100 calories; 128 grams carbohydrate; 92 grams protein; 29 grams fat; and 47 grams fiber.

BOOST FAT-BURNING WITH EXERCISE

You can follow this approach to eating—or any diet, for that matter—and lose weight, at least for a time. But you will be so much more successful, especially over the long haul, if you add regular exercise to the weight-loss equation. Here are some guidelines for accelerating your weight loss through exercise:

* Start out slowly, with an easy-to-do activity such as walking. Aim for three to five hours a week.

* After two to three weeks, begin to gradually increase the amount of effort you put in. You can do this by increasing the duration of your exercise session, say from 30 minutes to 45 minutes. The longer you work out, the more fat you'll burn. Or you can increase the number of times you work out each week. If you've been exercising three times a week, gradually work up to four or five times a week. You'll burn more calories—and more fat.

* Add a strength-training component, such as weight training, to your workout. Weight training builds body-shaping muscle and, because muscle is the body's most metabolically active tissue, increasing it helps burn more fat. Weight training also preserves lean muscle, which can wither away when you diet.

* Perform "combination exercise." This involves a single workout session in which you perform strength training, followed by some form of aerobic activity. This sequence—weight training first, aerobic activity second—shifts your body into a fat-burning mode. Lifting weights naturally forces your body to draw on stored muscle glycogen for fuel. During a 30- to 45-minute training session, you can use up a lot of glycogen. Afterward, your body is glycogen-needy—the perfect time to start your aerobics. Theoretically, your body then starts drawing on fatty acids for energy during the aerobics. You'll burn more fat, and get more trim as a result.

ENJOY THE RESULTS

After several weeks of eating and exercising according to this plan, you'll be slimmer, stronger, and healthier. And you will do it without sacrificing carbohydrates. When you reach your goal weight, gradually add carbohydrates back into your diet so you reach the 200-gram-a-day requirement. But always choose good carbs, using the scorecards in chapter 2. As for calories, research indicates that women can maintain their weight with a daily caloric intake of 1,400 to 1,900 calories a day; men, 2,000 to 2,500 calories or more, depending on activity levels. Your best bets for keeping your weight off include exercising on a regular basis and selecting natural, unprocessed high-fiber carbs in amounts that will keep unhealthy, excess pounds banished for good.

TEN

Carb Power for Exercisers and Athletes

If you are an exerciser or athlete, your goal is to maxi-mize your stamina, energy, and performance in order to be the very best you can be in your particular sport or physical endeavor. What is the optimum way to achieve that goal? In a word, carbohydrates. The key to push-yourself-to-the-limit performance lies in your body's chief energy fuel, carbohydrates.

The power of carbohydrates to improve stamina and boost performance has been known for well over a cen-tury. In fact, the carbohydrate/athletics story began as far back as 1887, when two French scientists observed that the jaw muscle of a horse rapidly took up glucose when the animal began chewing its food. In other words, the glucose gunned the horse's muscle. The rest, as they say, is history. Since then, carbohydrates have been considered the most important source of energy for fueling the active body. Consider the following:

- When you work out intensely during exercise, training, or competition, carbohydrates supply 80 to 95 percent of the fuel you burn.

- Unless your body is well stocked with carbohydrates, it will break down its own muscle for energy, and you will loss muscle mass, strength, and power.

- If you do not consume enough carbohydrates during exercise, your performance will slow down by as much as 60 percent of your normal capacity.

- As the primary fuel for your brain and nervous system, adequate carbohydrates give you the nutritional wherewithal to make quick decisions and fast reactions—both necessary to excellent performance in competitive athletics.

Like a gas tank with its limited number of gallons, your body has a limited capacity to store carbohydrates. Your muscles, for example, can store about 1,200 calories of glycogen; your liver, about 400 calories. If there were no other fuel source available during exercise (like fat), carbohydrates would provide enough nutritional "gas" for a 32-kilometer run, or about 20 miles. Thus, you must be diligent about refilling your body with sufficient carbohydrates. If you do so, you can train harder on successive workouts for greater gains.

The amount of glycogen you have in your muscular tanks is directly related to how much carbohydrate you eat and how well trained you are. Highly trained athletes, for example, are very efficient at storing muscle glycogen. Naturally, the more glycogen you can store in your muscles, the longer you can train or work out. So to achieve peak physical performance if you are an athlete or a serious exerciser, your diet should be higher in good carbs (at least 65 to 70 percent of your total daily calories) than what is recommended for less-active people. That being the case, let's look at specific carbohydrate strategies you should follow to ensure winning performance.

STRATEGY #1: STAY WELL FUELED WITH CARBOHYDRATES

To keep your muscles stocked with glycogen, stay on a carb-plentiful diet from week to week, one that is designed mostly with the many good carbs we have discussed throughout this book. This is the best, all-around strategy to follow for consistently high performance. Case in point: A study of hockey players, whose sport requires both muscular strength and aerobic endurance, found that during a three-day period between games, a high-carb diet caused a 45 percent higher glycogen refill than a diet lower in carbs. By consistently fueling yourself with carbs, you can keep your muscles well stocked with glycogen.

What counts as a high-carb athletic diet? Exercise scientists recommend that if you are a hard-training exerciser or athlete, you should eat between 7 and 8 grams of carbohydrates per kilograms of bodyweight on a daily basis to keep your glycogen tanks full.

Let's say, for example, that you weigh 150 pounds. In kilograms, your weight would be 68 kilograms (150 divided by 2.2). Thus, your daily carbohydrate intake should be 476 to 544 grams (68 times 7 or 8). Again, that means about 65 to 70 percent of your total daily caloric intake should come from carbs.

STRATEGY #2: PRACTICE "CARBOHYDRATE-LOADING" PRIOR TO COMPETITION

Used in competitive sports for more than thirty years, carbohydrate-loading is a technique of pushing more glycogen into your muscles than is normally available. Followed seven days prior to competition, carbohydrate-loading works best for endurance competitions lasting at least 60 to 90 minutes or more.

The scientifically accepted strategy for carbohydrate loading is as follows:

* Seven days prior to your competitive event, purposely empty your glycogen stores with an intense training bout that lasts approximately 90 minutes.

* Over the next three days, consume a varied, mixed diet composed of 45 to 50 percent carbohydrates. Train at moderate intensities for 45 to 60 minutes. (For an example of how to plan a precompetition meal, see the following table.)

* During the last three days prior to the competition, increase your carbohydrate intake to 70 percent of your total daily calories. Train at moderate intensities for 30 to 45 minutes. (Refer to the precompetition meal plan in the following table.)

* Two to four hours prior to the race, consume a high-carbohydrate meal. Ideally, eat about 100 to 200 grams of carbs, or roughly 400 to 800 calories. Choose solid or liquid foods, depending on what your system can best handle. Some examples include a combination of fruit, bread, rice, or pasta, with skim milk or nonfat yogurt. Other excellent prerace carbs include liquid meal replacers such as Boost or Ensure, or a product like GatorLode, a high-carbohydrate-loading source. GatorLode and similar products are formulated with carbohydrates only (no protein) and some vitamins. Be sure to drink 16 ounces of fluid two hours prior to your race to make sure you start the competition in a well-hydrated state.

PRECOMPETITION DIET PLANS

	45 to 50% Carbohydrates	70% Carbohydrates
Breakfast	1 slice whole-wheat toast 3 egg whites, scrambled 1 cup fresh blueberries 1 cup low-fat milk	1 cup Cream of Wheat cereal 1 cup low-fat milk 2 medium bran muffins ½ grapefruit
Snack	1 high-protein bar	1 cup fruit-flavored yogurt
Lunch	4 ounces cooked reduced-fat ham Potato salad: 1 medium boiled potato, 1 small celery stalk (chopped), 2 tablespoons low-fat mayonnaise, and 1 teaspoon yellow mustard 1 medium apple	Tuna sandwich: 2 ounces water-packed tuna, 2 slices whole-wheat bread, and 2 tablespoons low-fat mayonnaise 2 medium carrots 1 banana
Snack	1 cup fruit-flavored yogurt	1 sports bar containing carbohydrates and protein
Dinner	5 ounces grilled salmon 1 cup steamed and chopped broccoli 2 cups tossed salad 2 tablespoons reduced-calorie dressing	2 cups whole-wheat pasta 1 cup spaghetti sauce with 4 ounces cooked extra-lean ground turkey 2 cups tossed salad 2 tablespoons reduced-calorie dressing 1 cup fruit cocktail, water-packed ½ cup frozen nonfat yogurt

STRATEGY #3: INCORPORATE CARBOHYDRATE SUPPLEMENTS INTO YOUR DIET

Your personal fitness and training program should allow for the use of carbohydrate supplements. These include sports drinks with added electrolytes; carbohydrate meal replacers formulated with protein; and sports bars containing carbohydrates, proteins, and other nutrients. Carbohydrate supplements like these are designed to replenish nutrients lost during exercise, provide energy, or enhance muscle growth. Further, the performance-enhancing advantages of these supplements are backed by impressive research. Some of the most popular and effective carbohydrate supplements are discussed in the following sections.

Sports Drinks (Fluid-Replacers)

Also known as fluid-replacers, these beverages contain mostly water (about 85 percent), but are formulated with electrolytes and small amounts of carbohydrates. Electrolytes are dissolved minerals; their job in your body is to conduct electrical charges that let them react with other minerals to relay nerve impulses, make muscles contract or relax, and help carry water through the small intestine and into the bloodstream. Electrolytes can be lost through sweat during hard workouts, athletic competitions lasting an hour or longer, or heavy on-the-job physical labor, and need to be replenished.

Sports drinks do a number of things: They supply energy for working muscles, enhance performance, stimulate rapid fluid absorption, encourage better fluid consumption due to their sweet taste, and replace water and electrolytes lost through sweat.

Most sports drinks are formulated with about 6 to 8 percent carbohydrates. The main forms of carbohydrates used in these supplements are glucose, fructose, and sucrose—a combination shown in research to be very effective at accelerating energy to your muscles.

Fructose, however, isn't as fast at furnishing muscle glycogen as glucose is. What's more, fructose can cause digestive problems if it is the only carbohydrate used in a sports drink. Even so, fructose is beneficial in promoting rapid resynthesis of liver glycogen. That's important, too, because whereas muscles tap into their own private stock of glycogen for energy, the liver stores glycogen for use by the entire body. This is one case in which fructose earns respect as a good carb.

Sports drinks are very safe when used as directed. It is best to avoid products that are carbonated or that contain caffeine. Carbonated beverages release their carbonation (carbon dioxide) in the stomach, which increases the risk of bloating, stomachache, and nausea. Caffeine acts as a diuretic, which can be detrimental during endurance competition.

Carbohydrate Meal-Replacers

Available as bars, in cans, or mix-it-yourself powders, meal-replacers are formulated to reproduce as closely as possible the nutrition you would get from food, complete with carbohydrates, protein, fat, vitamins, and minerals.

Meal-replacers serve as fortified snacks, as a supplement to a healthy diet, and as a performance-enhancing food used most effectively post-workout to aid in muscle recovery. Unlike sports drinks, they contain a higher amount of carbohydrates, usually about 60 grams or so. Meal-replacers are not to be confused with "carbohydrate-loaders," a type of liquid supplement formulated with only carbohydrates and no protein.

As to which is better for an endurance athlete, bar or beverage, it depends on personal choice. Beverages are great if you can't tolerate solids before or following exercise. Bars, on the other hand, have advantages in certain sports, such as long-distance cycling. Many cyclists like to wrap taffylike meal-replacer bars around their handlebars. The bars stick without crumbling, and the cyclists can simply peel them off and munch when needed.

Because these products vary in nutrient composition, try several brands to determine which works best for you. Never test-drive a new product at competition time; instead, experiment through trial and error during training.

Don't use meal-replacers in lieu of real meals to skimp on calories, at least not on a regular basis. They really aren't intended for that purpose, despite their name. Meal-replacers fail to provide all the nutritious food factors such as disease-preventing phytochemicals found in actual food. If you're dieting and want to use a meal-replacer as a snack, be sure to figure in its calorie count in your daily allowance. Most of these products contain between 250 and 350 calories per serving.

Energy Gels

Energy gels are highly concentrated carbohydrates with a puddinglike consistency that are packaged in single-serve pouches. Designed for athletes and exercisers, these products provide 70 to 100 calories and 17 to 25 grams carbohydrates per serving. The carbohydrate source is usually a mixture of simple carbs (usually fructose or dextrose) and maltodextrin or cornstarch. Some of the leading products on the market include ReLode, Clif Hot Shot, Pocket Rocket, and Squeezy.

Quickly absorbed into the bloodstream, energy gels are a good source of immediate food energy, particularly during extended exercise efforts. Experts generally advise that if you're an endurance athlete, you need to refuel yourself during exercise with 50 to 60 grams carbohydrates each hour. That being so, take one energy gel packet every 30 minutes during a long race, bicycle ride, or other endurance event.

These supplements generally contain no fiber or other nutrients and, therefore, should not be used to replace the good carbs in your diet. When using energy gels, make sure you take in sufficient water to process the carbohydrates and prevent dehydration.

SUPPLEMENTAL RIBOSE

What It Is: Supplemental ribose is a relatively new supplement available in tablets, nutritional drinks, energy bars, or in powder form. It may help boost your pep by revving up certain energy-producing systems in your body. Ribose occurs naturally in your body anyway, and so taking in some extra may give you an edge.

For background, your body's own ribose is found in every cell. It is a beneficial simple sugar that forms the backbone of DNA and RNA, the genetic material that controls cellular growth and reproduction.

Ribose stimulates your body's production of ATP (adenosine triphosphate), the main energy-releasing molecule of all living cells. Cells need ATP to function properly. Your heart uses ATP to beat, for example, and your muscles use it to move.

Normally, your body can produce and recycle all the ATP it needs, especially when there is an abundant supply of oxygen. But under certain circumstances—namely ischemia (lack of blood flow to tissues) and strenuous exercise—ATP cannot be regenerated fast enough, and energy-producing compounds called adenine nucleotides may be lost from cells. This can impair muscle function and tax strength, because cells need adenine nucleotides to produce sufficient amounts of ATP.

Proof that intense exercise can deplete cells of energy-producing nucleotides was demonstrated dramatically in a study published in the *Journal of Applied Physiology* in which eleven healthy men engaged in high-intensity training on a cycle ergometer three times a week for six weeks, then afterward trained twice a day for a week. Another group (nine men) rested for six weeks, then trained twice a day with the others. In the first group, nucleotide content of skeletal muscle dropped by 13 percent; in the second group, by 25 percent. In both groups, nucleotide levels had not fully recovered even after seventy-two hours of rest.

Ribose supplementation may restore these lost nucleotides. In one animal study, ribose supplementation increased the rate of nucleotide synthesis in resting and exercising muscles by three to four times. Other animal studies have found that ribose can restore energy levels to near normal within twelve to twenty-four hours. Studies are ongoing to confirm that ribose may be equally as beneficial in humans.

To preserve high cellular levels of ATP, the recommended dosage of supplemental ribose is 3 to 5 grams daily as maintenance dose, and 5 to 10 grams daily if you are a competitive athlete.

Ribose supplements appear to be safe, although at mega doses (60 grams a day), it causes gastrointestinal problems. If you have a heart condition or other serious medical problem, consult your physician before supplementing.

Wise Use of Carbohydrate Supplements

Always think of these products as supplements, or additions, to your diet, rather than substitutes for wholesome, natural carbs. Ultimately, the best way to fuel and nourish your body is by eating a varied, nutrient-rich diet of low-fat proteins and dairy products, fruits, grains, and vegetables.

STRATEGY #4: TIME YOUR USE OF CARBOHYDRATES, INCLUDING SUPPLEMENTS

As critical as the amount and type of carbohydrates you consume is the timing of your intake. There are three critical periods in which to consider consuming carbohydrates: before your workout, during your workout, and after your workout.

Preworkout: If you're an endurance athlete, use carbohydrate meal-replacers as pre-exercise snacks to boost calories for extra energy. You can also use meal-replacers for carbohydrate-loading, in addition to other carb sources, to keep your glycogen reserves well stocked for competition.

If you're a strength trainer in a mass-building phase and want to push to the max, fuel yourself with carbohydrates before your workout. Eat a low-fat, high-carb meal two to three hours prior to working out. In addition, make sure you are always well hydrated and drink 4 to 8 ounces of fluid immediately before exercise. Following this pattern will ensure you gain the greatest energy advantage from your pre-exercise meal without feeling full while you exercise.

Liquid meal replacers are a terrific pre-exercise carb choice. In a study of strength trainers, one group consumed a carbohydrate drink just before training. Another group was given a placebo. For exercise, both groups did leg extensions at about 80 percent of their strength capacity, performing repeated sets of 10 repetitions with rest between sets. What the researchers found was that the carbohydrate-fed group outlasted the placebo group, performing many more sets and repetitions.

During your workout: If you want a little extra boost to improve your endurance during training or competition, supplement with a sports drink (like Gatorade) during your workout. For example, sip a half-cup of a sports drink every fifteen to twenty minutes to extend your endurance. This helps stabilize your blood sugar levels and maintain fluid levels and gives you extra pep. Research has consistently shown that drinking a sports drink during competition delays fatigue. By supplementing with a sports drink during competition, you spare your existing muscle and liver glycogen stores. That means you can run, bike, or swim longer because you're fueling yourself with a supplemental source of carbs so your body doesn't run out of steam.

Strength trainers can also benefit from a carb boost during training. Case in point: In one study, exercisers drank either a placebo or a 10 percent carbohydrate sports drink immediately prior to and between the fifth, tenth, fifteenth sets of a strength training workout. They performed repeated sets of ten repetitions, with three minutes of rest between each set. When fueled by the carb drink, they could do more total repetitions than when they drank the placebo, which all goes to show that carbs clearly give you an energy edge when consumed during a workout. The harder you can work out, the more you can stimulate your muscles to grow.

But if you're trying to lose body fat, you might want to forgo supplemental carbs during your workouts, because although carbs boost your power and stamina, they might keep your body from dipping into its fat reserves for energy. Your entire workout could be powered solely on carb fuel and never significantly tap into fat stores for fuel. By working out in a moderately carb-needy state (no preworkout carbs), you can theoretically force your body to start using more fat for fuel. The downside, though, is that you could run low on energy.

The key here is to consider your goals—mass-building or fat-burning—and listen to your body for signs of fatigue. Adjust your carb intake accordingly, depending on your goals and energy levels.

Be sure to have a sports drink handy if you're exercising or working in hot weather, too. That's when fluid loss is greater than any other time of the year. You can lose more electrolytes, too, although the concentration of these minerals in sweat gets weaker the fitter you are. You also burn more glycogen working out in the heat—another good reason to quench your body with a sports drink.

Post-workout: You've just finished a super-intense

workout. If you could zoom down to the microscopic level of your muscles, you'd be astounded by the sight. There are tears in the tiny structures of your muscle fibers and leaks in muscle cells. Inflammation is setting in, and like cellular medics, white blood cells are on the scene to mend the damage and fix the leaks. Over the next twenty-four to forty-eight hours, muscle protein will break down, and additional muscle glycogen will be used up.

These are some of the chief metabolic events that occur in the aftermath of a hard workout. And although they might look like havoc, these events are actually a necessary part of "recovery"—the repair and growth of muscle tissue that take place after every workout.

During recovery, your body replenishes muscle glycogen and synthesizes new muscle protein. In the process, muscle fibers are made bigger and stronger to protect themselves against future trauma. Actual muscle growth occurs not while you're exercising, but in the recovery period following your workout.

There is much you can do to enhance this recovery process, and carbohydrates are a must-have, because your muscles are most receptive to producing new glycogen within the first few hours following your workout. This is the period in which blood flow to your muscles is much greater, a condition that makes muscle cells thirsty for glucose. Muscle cells are also more sensitive to the effects of insulin during this time, and insulin promotes glycogen restoration. Therefore, consume carbs *immediately* after you work out. Canned meal-replacers or sports bars are an easy way to immediately refuel.

Continue to take in 50 to 100 grams of carbohydrate every two hours following your workout until you resume your normal meal patterns. Strive for a total intake of 600 grams from food and supplements within twenty-four hours after your workout.

Another benefit of this post-training snack is that it

helps trigger the elevation of key hormones (insulin and growth hormone) involved in muscle growth, especially in the period right after exercise. Case in point: At the University of Texas in Austin, nine experienced male strength trainers were given either water (which served as the control), a carbohydrate supplement, a protein supplement, or a carbohydrate/protein supplement.

The subjects took their designated supplement immediately after working out and again two hours later. Right after exercise and throughout the next eight hours, the researchers drew blood samples to determine the levels of various hormones in the blood, including insulin, testosterone (a male hormone also involved in muscle growth), and growth hormone.

The most significant finding was that the carbohydrate/protein supplement triggered the greatest elevations in insulin and growth hormone. Clearly, protein works hand in hand with post-exercise carbs to create a hormonal environment that's highly conducive to muscle growth.

For building muscle, consume a meal-replacer with your meals to boost calories. It takes an additional 2,500 calories a week to manufacture a pound of muscle. Increasing your calories by about 350 a day with a meal-replacer is an effective way to achieve that caloric surplus.

STRATEGY #5: SELECT MOSTLY FAST-FUELING CARBOHYDRATES

The best types of carbs for refueling are those with a moderate- to high-glycemic index (GI) rating. These carbohydrates are digested and absorbed more rapidly, resulting in faster glycogen resynthesis. Such carbs include sports drinks, meal-replacers (beverages or bars), bagels, potatoes, brown rice, raisins, corn, sweet potatoes, oatmeal, and oranges.

A word of caution: There is a drawback of high-glycemic index foods. They might produce a fast, undesirable surge of blood sugar. When this happens, the pancreas responds by oversecreting insulin to remove sugar from the blood. Blood sugar then drops to a too-low level, and you can feel weak or dizzy.

Low-glycemic index foods, on the other hand, provide a more constant release of energy and are unlikely to lead to these reactions. By mixing and matching low- and high-glycemic foods in your diet, you can keep your blood sugar levels stable from meal to meal. The watchword here is *moderation:* Don't overdose on high-glycemic index foods or beverages.

STAY CARB-CHARGED

*Whatever your sport or exercise, the single most impor-*tant dietary factor affecting your performance is the amount of carbohydrates in your daily diet. Eating a high-carbohydrate diet, with mostly good carbs, will keep your muscles well fueled so you can challenge yourself physically and improve your performance during your regular workouts. Stick with good carbs as the mainstay of your diet, and you won't believe how great you'll look and how strong you'll feel.

PART III

Special Topics

ELEVEN

Your Smart-Carb Strategy

When you really think about it, deciding which carbs to eat boils down to some basic common sense: The more natural a carb is, the better it is for your body, because your body uses pure, natural carbs so much more efficiently than it uses processed junk carbs. Pure carbs are bursting with nutrients, each put to use in building and healing the body. Processed carbs, on the other hand, are nutritionally bankrupt and associated with various health problems.

So the key is to make carb choices that make sense for your particular situation, for example: Does diabetes run in your family, or are you struggling with it now? Do you want to do everything you can to deter cancer? Has your doctor told you to manage your digestive health with a higher-fiber diet? Do you have high triglycerides or cholesterol? Do you need to lose weight? Are you an athlete who wants to enhance performance naturally? Are you suffering from a health problem that might be helped with good carbs?

Once you've answered these questions, you can begin

an overhaul of your nutrition program in order to eat more healthfully. Depending on your personal health and fitness goals, you will require a certain amount of carbohydrates each day—usually 40, 55, or 65 percent of your total daily calories. You can easily compute your allotment using the following formula:

> Multiply your *total daily calories* by *the percentage of total daily calories from carbs* divided by *4,* the number of grams in each gram of carbohydrate, to determine your *daily carb requirements* in grams.

Let's suppose, for example, that you want to determine your carbohydrate needs for a 2,000-calorie diet in which 65 percent of your calories come from carbs. Here's how the calculation works out:

- Multiply your total daily calories by 65 percent (.65). For example: 2,000 calories × .65 = 1,300.
- Divide your daily carb calories by 4, the number of grams in each gram of carbohydrate: 1,300 ÷ 4 = 325 grams total carbohydrate for the day.

To make it even easier, I've included the following table, which lists amounts of carbs in grams for various caloric levels and percentages. You'll also find a table listing the carb count for many of the carbs discussed in this book.

Caloric Level	Total Carb Grams in a 40% Carb Diet	Total Carb Grams in a 55% Carb Diet	Total Carb Grams in a 65% Carb Diet
1,200	120 grams	165 grams	195 grams
1,500	150 grams	206 grams	244 grams
1,800	180 grams	248 grams	293 grams
2,000	200 grams	275 grams	325 grams
2,200	220 grams	303 grams	358 grams
2,500	250 grams	344 grams	406 grams
3,000	300 grams	413 grams	488 grams

	Food	Serving Size	Carbohydrates (grams)
Beverages	Apple juice	1 cup	21
	Carrot juice	1 cup	22
	Concord grape juice	1 cup	32
	Cranberry juice cocktail	1 cup	14
	Grapefruit juice	1 cup	23
	Pineapple juice	1 cup	29
	Tomato juice	1 cup	9
Breads	Bagel	1 medium	38
	Bran muffin	1 medium	18
	Branola (high-fiber)	1 slice	18
	Pita pocket	1 whole	31
	Pumpernickel bread	1 slice	10
	Rye bread	1 slice	10
	Stone-Ground whole-wheat bread	1 slice	14
	Whole-wheat bread	1 slice	12

(continued)

	Food	Serving Size	Carbohydrates (grams)
Cereals	100% Bran	⅓ cup	23
	All Bran	½ cup	23
	All-Bran with Extra Fiber	½ cup	23
	Bran Chex	1 cup	39
	Fiber One	½ cup	24
	Granola	¾ cup	36
	Raisin Bran	1 cup	47
	Shredded Wheat and Bran	1 ¼ cup	47
	Special K	1 cup	23
	Oat bran, cooked	½ cup	41
	Oatmeal	½ cup	14
Dairy Foods	Low-fat milk	1 cup	11
	Skim milk	1 cup	13
	Yogurt, sugar free	1 cup	14
Diabetic Supplements	Choice DM bar	1 bar	19
	Choice DM beverage	8 ounces	24
	Glucerna bar	1 bar	24
	Glucerna beverage	8 ounces	29
Fruits	Apple	1 medium	21
	Apricots, dried	6 halves	12
	Avocado	1 medium	15
	Banana	1 medium	28
	Blueberries	1 cup	20
	Cantaloupe	1 medium wedge	6
	Cherries	1 cup	70
	Figs, dried	2 figs	24
	Grapefruit	½ fruit	9
	Grapes	1 cup	16
	Kiwifruit	1 medium	11
	Orange	1 medium	15

(continued)

	Food	Serving Size	Carbohydrates (grams)
Fruits	Papaya	1 whole	30
	Peach	1 medium	11
	Pear	1 medium	25
	Pineapple	1 cup chunks	19
	Plum	1 medium	9
	Prunes, stewed	1 cup	69
	Raspberries	1 cup	51
	Strawberries	1 cup	11
Legumes, Cooked	Black beans	½ cup	17
	Garbanzo beans	½ cup	17
	Kidney beans	½ cup	20
	Lentils	½ cup	13
	Lima beans	½ cup	20
	Navy beans	½ cup	17
	Peas	½ cup	12
	Pinto beans	½ cup	15
	Soy milk	1 cup	4
	Soybeans	½ cup	8
	Tofu	2 ounces	1
Pasta	Macaroni	½ cup	18
	Whole-wheat spaghetti	½ cup	18
Sports Supplements	Gatorade	8 ounces	14
	GatorLode (Hi-Carb)	11.6 ounces	71
	PowerBar	1 bar	28
Vegetables	Artichoke, boiled	1 cup	19
	Beets, boiled	1 cup	17
	Broccoli, boiled	1 cup	8
	Broccoli sprouts	1 cup	10
	Cabbage, boiled	1 cup	7

(continued)

	Food	Serving Size	Carbohydrates (grams)
Vegetables	Carrot	1 medium, raw	6
	Corn, canned	1 cup	19
	Onions, raw	¼ cup, chopped	3
	Potato, baked	1 medium	51
	Red pepper, raw	¼ cup, chopped	2
	Romaine lettuce, raw	1 cup	2
	Spinach, boiled	1 cup	7
	Sweet potato, baked	1 medium	28
	Tomato, raw	1 medium	6
	Winter squash, baked	1 cup	30
Whole Grains	Brown rice	½ cup	21
	Bulgur wheat	½ cup	24
	Couscous	½ cup	18
	Quinoa	½ cup	58
	Wheat bran	2 table-spoons	4

In the following sections are several health scenarios that sum up specific carbohydrate recommendations for certain situations and conditions. Use them as general guidelines and customize them where necessary. Some of this information has been covered in previous chapters, but is repeated here to give you a quick summary for review.

GOOD-CARB GUIDELINES FOR BRAIN FITNESS

Carbohydrates are the leading nutrient fuel for your brain, supplying glucose for mental alertness, a bright mood, and a sharp memory. A brain-healthy diet should supply 55 to 65 percent of its total daily calories from good carbs. Most of these carbs should come from fruits and vegetables (at least five servings a day), because these foods are rich in antioxidants and phytochemicals, both of which protect brain cells from damage.

GOOD-CARB GUIDELINES FOR PREVENTING CANCER

Eating a healthy diet is one of the most significant moves you can make to prevent cancer. Generally, your diet should supply:

- 55 to 65 percent of total daily calories from good carbs
- 25 to 35 grams of fiber daily

In addition, the American Cancer Society recommends the following nutritional guidelines:

- Choose most of the foods you eat from plant sources. These include fiber-rich carbs such as fruits, vegetables, whole grains, and legumes. These foods are packed with vitamins, minerals, antioxidants, and phytochemicals—all known to reduce your risk of cancer. Eat at least five servings a day of fruits and vegetables; this amount has been shown in scientific research to reduce the risk of cancer, particularly lung cancer and colon cancer.

- Limit your intake of high-fat foods, especially those from animal sources. High-fat diets are tied to an increased risk of cancers of the colon, rectum, prostate, and endometrium.

- Stay physically active and maintain a healthy weight. Exercising thirty or more minutes a day helps control your weight (obesity is a risk factor for cancer), cuts your odds of colon cancer, and helps enhance your overall health.

• Limit or avoid drinking alcoholic beverages. Drinking alcohol increases your risk of cancer of the mouth, esophagus, pharynx, larynx, and liver in men and women and breast cancer in women.

GOOD-CARB GUIDELINES FOR DIABETES

Diabetes is a complex disease, requiring treatment that involves diet, exercise, lifestyle adjustments, and, for many people, injectable insulin or oral diabetes drugs. Generally, the recommended diet is one that is moderate in good carbs, low in saturated fat, and high in fiber. This translates into:

• 40 to 55 percent of total daily calories from good carbs

• 25 to 35 grams of fiber daily

If you have diabetes, you should eat less sugar. Foods high in sugar include desserts, sugar breakfast cereals, candy, table sugar, honey, syrup, and soft drinks. Generally, 10 percent or less of your total daily calories should come from added sugar.

The timing of your meals is also very important for preventing hypoglycemia (low blood sugar) and feeling energetic. Therefore, eat multiple meals and snacks, and try to spread those meals throughout the day. It's best to try to space your major meals four to five hours apart, and leave two hours between meals and snacks to allow for adequate digestion. Your body works best when nutrients are replenished every few hours.

In addition, be consistent on when you eat and how

much you eat. Eat meals and snacks at approximately the same time every day, and eat the same portion sizes each day. This will help you achieve a balance among food, medication, and activity.

If you have type II diabetes, concentrate on cutting fat in your diet, particularly saturated fat and cholesterol, as well as losing weight, because a high-fat diet is a risk factor for heart disease, the major complication of diabetes.

The same dietary strategies, namely the selection of good carbs in carefully controlled amounts, that are used to manage diabetes can also be employed to prevent it.

GOOD-CARB GUIDELINES FOR DIGESTIVE HEALTH

The number-one recommendation for excellent digestive health is to eat a high-fiber diet, with 25 to 35 grams, or more, of fiber from good carbs. Because of its ability to add bulk to the diet and softness to the stool, fiber moves through your digestive system like a one-nutrient janitorial crew, cleaning out toxins, cancer-causing agents, and cholesterol. This attribute earns fiber its reputation for being the most effective remedy for constipation, as well as for reducing the risk of many serious digestive diseases, including diverticulosis and colon cancer. The best high-fiber carbs are beans, legumes, whole grains, fiber-fortified cereals, and certain fruits.

GOOD-CARB GUIDELINES FOR HEART DISEASE

To bring your triglycerides and cholesterol down, your carbohydrate intake should be 55 to 60 percent of your total daily calories. (This is the carb intake recommended for heart health by the American Heart Association.)

It is preferable to choose good carbs—vegetables, fruits, whole grains, and high-fiber cereals—over simple sugars. Good carbs supply more fiber, vitamins, minerals, antioxidants, and phytochemicals than foods high in added sugars. Research has shown that sugar might be a risk factor for heart disease because it elevates triglycerides, which are harmful to the heart. Thus, avoid products that list more than 5 grams of sugar per serving on the label. If the specific amount of sugar is unlisted, shun products with sugar listed as one of the first four ingredients on the label. Sugar goes by various other names, too: sucrose, dextrose, maltose, lactose, maltodextrin, corn syrup, and high-fructose corn syrup, to name just a few.

Strive to eat five or more daily servings of fruits and vegetables, and six or more servings of grains—bread, cereal, or rice, for example.

Other recommendations include the following:

• Restrict your fat intake to 30 percent of your total calories. Less than 7 percent of your total calories should come from saturated fats and fats called trans fats, which are found in stick margarine and vegetable shortening.

• Limit your daily intake of dietary cholesterol to less than 200 milligrams.

• Exercise for thirty or more minutes most days of the week.

If your triglycerides and cholesterol don't change for the better with diet and exercise, consult your physician. You might need a prescription medication to normalize your blood fats.

GOOD-CARB GUIDELINES FOR WEIGHT CONTROL

Being overweight, defined as 20 percent or more above your ideal weight, puts you in harm's way of numerous life-threatening diseases, among them heart problems, stroke, cancer, and diabetes.

Without question, it can be challenging to lose weight, especially if you're far from your ideal weight. But it's not impossible, either.

One of the most important steps you can take is to choose mainly good carbs in the following amounts:

* 40 percent of your total daily calories from good carbs (This amount is low enough to encourage your body to burn stored fat.)

* 120 to 150 grams a day of good carbs

* 25 to 35 grams of fiber daily (Eating 35 grams of fiber a day is most effective for reducing body fat.)

In addition, eat fewer calories than your body uses each day. To lose 1 pound of body fat, you have to create a 3,500-calorie deficit, either by eating less, exercising more, or both. By cutting your total calorie intake by 500 calories each day, for example, you should be able to lose 1 pound a week (500 calories × 7 days)—a safe rate of weight loss. If you add exercise to this equation and burn any extra calories, your fat loss will be even greater. An hour of exercise, for example, can burn up anywhere from 250 to 500 calories.

Your weight-loss diet should be as low in fat as possible, because reducing dietary fat is one of the best ways to shed pounds. By keeping your total fat intake to 30 percent or less of your total daily calories, you might be able to lose body fat with less restriction in total calories.

In addition, try to curb your intake of fat-forming foods such as sugar, processed foods, and alcohol. By limiting these foods, you'll automatically reduce the number of calories in your diet.

GOOD-CARB GUIDELINES FOR ATHLETIC PERFORMANCE

Ideally, 60 to 65 percent of the calories in your daily diet should come from carbohydrates, particularly good carbs, and this requirement goes for most physically active people. The best way to increase good carbohydrates is to add foods like whole grains, whole-grain cereals and breads, potatoes, yams, and legumes to your diet. Feel free to use higher-glycemic carbs, such as sports drinks, to refuel and restock your muscles with glycogen for energy. Other carbohydrate supplements, such as those discussed in chapter 10, are useful for enhancing performance, endurance, and muscle growth.

GOOD CARBS FOR LIFE

*As you read through these guidelines, you probably de-*tected a single thread running through each: Natural, unprocessed good carbs—grains, vegetables, and fruits—are healthy for every part of your body. Put another way, what is good for your brain is good for your heart—and for practically every other organ and body system. Good carbs simply mean good health.

TWELVE

Good-Carb Cooking

Now that you know good carbs will get you on the road to good health, what's the next step? Start cooking with them and incorporating them into your daily diet. With so many good carbs available, you can have a field day in your kitchen. What you will find here are thirty-two good-carb recipes for every possible course, from dips to desserts. Each of these recipes has been tested by the organizations that created them and use many of the very best carbs discussed in this book. *Bon appetit!*

DIPS

Avo Salsa

2 ripe medium California avocados, peeled, pitted, and diced

1 large ripe tomato, diced

¼ cup finely chopped red onion

2 cloves garlic, minced

2 tablespoons chopped fresh cilantro

Juice of 1 large lime

½ teaspoon ground cumin

½ teaspoon freshly ground black pepper

½ teaspoon salt

1. In a medium bowl, combine avocados, tomato, onion, garlic, cilantro, lime juice, cumin, pepper and salt.
2. Toss well and maintain chunky consistency.

Serves 8.
Reprinted with permission from the California Avocado Commission, www.avocado.org.

◆ ◆ ◆

California Avocado Green Onion Dip

1 medium California avocado, seeded and peeled

1 tablespoon fresh lemon juice

1 cup 1 percent low-fat cottage cheese

¾ cup plain nonfat yogurt

¼ **cup nonfat mayonnaise**

4 green onions, thinly sliced (about ½ cup)

¼ **cup carrots, shredded (about ½ medium carrot)**

1½ **cups broccoli florets**

1 cup cucumber slices

28 melba toast rounds

1. Dice avocado into small pieces, toss with lemon juice, and set aside.
2. In a food processor or blender, blend cottage cheese, yogurt, and mayonnaise until smooth.
3. Add cottage cheese mixture to avocado, gently stirring in onions and carrots.
4. Cover and chill. Serve with broccoli, cucumber, and melba toast, allowing ½ cup vegetables, 4 melba toast rounds, and 8 tablespoons dip per serving.

Serves 7.

Reprinted with permission from the California Avocado Commission, www.avocado.org

◆ ◆ ◆

Artichokes with Light Honey-Mustard Dip

4 medium California artichokes

½ **cup light mayonnaise**

2 teaspoons honey

½ **teaspoon mustard**

½ **teaspoon fresh lemon juice**

1. Wash artichokes under cold running water. Cut off stem at base; remove small bottom leaves. If de-

sired; trim tips of leaves and cut off top 2 inches. Stand artichokes upright in a deep, nonreactive saucepan large enough to hold snugly.

2. Add 1 teaspoon salt and 2 to 3 inches boiling water. Cover and boil gently 35 to 45 minutes or until avocado base can be pierced easily with a fork. (Add a little more boiling water, if needed.) Turn artichokes upside down to drain. Serve immediately or cool completely; cover and refrigerate to chill. Makes 4 artichokes.

3. Combine light mayonnaise, honey, mustard, and lemon juice; mix well.

_____

Makes about ¹/₂ cup.
Reprinted with permission from the California Artichoke Advisory Board, www.artichokes.org.

SOUPS

Boston Bean Soup

1 cup dried pinto beans, or 2 (15-ounce) cans cooked pinto beans, drained

2 medium tomatoes, seeded and chopped

1 rib celery, sliced

1 medium onion, chopped

1 bay leaf

1 (15-ounce) can reduced-sodium, fat-free beef broth

Salt and freshly ground black pepper to taste

1. If using canned beans, ignore this step. If using dried beans, place in a small Dutch casserole. Add

3 cups cold water. Cover and bring to a boil. Remove from heat and soak one hour. Drain well.

2. In a medium pan, mix together beans, tomatoes, celery, onion, bay leaf, and broth. Cover and bring to boil over medium-high heat. Reduce heat and simmer until vegetables are quite soft, 60 to 75 minutes for dried beans, 20 minutes for canned. Let hot soup sit, uncovered, 20 minutes. Remove bay leaf.

3. Purée half the soup in a blender. Recombine with remaining soup. Season to taste with salt and pepper.

_____

Makes 4 servings.
Reprinted with permission from the American Institute of Cancer Research, www.aicr.org.

◆ ◆ ◆

Kidney Bean and Quinoa Chowder

2 teaspoons olive oil

¾ cup chopped onion

1 rib celery, cut in ½-inch slices

¼ cup quinoa, rinsed well and drained

1 small zucchini, cut in ½-inch cubes

1 medium red or white potato, cut in ½-inch cubes

½ Granny Smith or Fuji apple, peeled, cored, and cut in
   ½-inch cubes

6 cups vegetable broth

1 (10-ounce) can kidney beans, drained and rinsed

1 cup fresh, frozen, or canned corn kernels

Salt and freshly ground pepper to taste

2 tablespoons chopped fresh cilantro, for garnish

1. Heat oil in a large saucepan over medium-high
   heat. Sauté onion and celery until onion is translucent, about 5 minutes.
2. Add quinoa, zucchini, potato, and apple. Pour in
   broth. Bring to a boil, reduce heat, and simmer
   until potatoes are tender and grain is cooked, about
   15 minutes.
3. Add beans and corn. Cook until heated through.
   Season chowder to taste with salt and pepper. Ladle
   into warm bowls, garnish with cilantro, and serve.

Makes 4 servings.

Variation: Along with beans and corn, add 1 to 2 corn tortillas, torn into bite-size pieces, or ¾ cup cubed cooked
chicken.

Cooking for two: This soup keeps two to three days in the refrigerator and reheats well. So take a break, then serve it again in a couple days. The second time, garnish with a squirt of fresh lime juice instead of cilantro.

Reprinted with permission from the American Institute of Cancer Research, www.aicr.org.

SALADS

Spinach Salad

1 pound spinach, torn into bite-size pieces
1 medium red onion, thinly sliced
1 small can mandarin oranges, drained
½ cup almonds

Combine spinach, onion, oranges, and almonds and serve with desired dressing.

Reprinted with permission from the Pioneer Valley Growers Association, www.pvga.net.

◆   ◆   ◆

Sweet Potato Salad

3 pound sweet potatoes

1½ cups nonfat plain yogurt

2 tablespoons fresh cilantro, minced

2 tablespoons shallots, minced

1 tablespoon fresh lime juice

Salt and freshly ground black pepper to taste

1 green bell pepper, seeded and chopped

2 celery stalks, chopped

Chopped canned chiles to taste

1. Preheat oven to 400 degrees.
2. Scrub sweet potatoes and pierce all over with a fork. Bake until soft, about 1 hour. While potatoes are baking, prepare dressing.
3. Make dressing by mixing together yogurt, cilantro, shallots, and lime juice. Add salt to taste. Chill at least 1 hour before using to dress salad.
4. When sweet potatoes are baked, cool, peel, and cut in ½-inch cubes. Place in large bowl and mix in salt and pepper to taste. Mix potatoes with bell pepper, celery, and chiles.
5. Mix dressing into potato salad. Serve warm or chilled.

Makes 6 servings.
Reprinted with permission from the American Institute of Cancer Research, www.aicr.org.

• • •

Curried Couscous Salad

1¼ cups fat-free, reduced-sodium chicken broth

1 tablespoon curry powder

1 tablespoon extra-virgin olive oil, divided

¾ cup couscous

½ cup carrot, cut in ½-inch dice

½ cup Spanish onion, cut in ½-inch dice

½ cup tomato, seeded and cut in ½-inch dice

½ cup zucchini, cut in ½-inch dice

¼ cup dried currants

2 tablespoons fresh lemon juice

Salt and freshly ground pepper to taste

1. In a medium saucepan over medium-high heat, combine broth, curry powder, and 2 teaspoons oil. Bring to a boil. Stir in couscous, reduce heat, cover, and cook 1 minute. Remove from heat and let couscous sit, covered, 10 minutes.
2. Fluff couscous with fork and pour into a large bowl. Stir in carrot, onion, tomato, zucchini, and currants.
3. In a small bowl, combine lemon juice, salt, and pepper. Whisk in remaining 1 teaspoon oil. Pour dressing over salad. Toss with fork until all ingredients are combined. Season to taste with salt. Serve warm or at room temperature.

Makes 6 servings.

Variation: Mix in ½ cup canned chickpeas or ½ cup shredded, cooked chicken breast.

Reprinted with permission from the American Institute of Cancer Research, www.aicr.org.

◆ ◆ ◆

Golden Fruit Salad

1 medium mango

1 Gala or Golden Delicious apple, peeled, cored, and thinly sliced

½ Asian pear, peeled, cored, and thinly sliced

1 peach or nectarine, thinly sliced

½ cup red seedless grapes, halved

6 whole dried apricots, or 9 halves, cut in ½-inch slivers

1 tablespoon finely chopped, candied or preserved ginger

½ cup orange juice

½ teaspoon vanilla

1. To cube mango, place on counter. Holding a knife horizontally, cut off one side of mango, slicing as close to pit as possible. Turn fruit over and repeat to remove other side. Hold one half in the palm of your hand, skin-side down. Using top of knife, score mango vertically and horizontally, making cuts about ¾ inch apart and slicing fruit so you feel tip of knife against skin of fruit. Grasp two opposite sides of fruit between your thumb and fingers and turn skin back so scored squares stand out like a porcupine's quills. Holding the knife horizontally, carefully cut cubes of mango at their base, separating them from skin. Place cubed fruit in a large serving bowl.
2. Add apple, Asian pear, peach or nectarine, grapes, and apricots to mango and toss gently to combine.

Add ginger, orange juice, and vanilla, then toss again.

3. Let fruit salad sit 15 minutes, at room temperature, so flavors can meld. Serve immediately or cover with plastic and refrigerate 3 to 4 hours. The fruit becomes mushy if left longer.

_____

Makes 6 to 8 servings.
Reprinted with permission from the American Institute of Cancer Research, www.aicr.org.

◆ ◆ ◆

Marinated Vegetable Salad

1 (16-ounce) package frozen California blend vegetables

½ cup sugar

1 tablespoon flour

1 teaspoon dry mustard

½ teaspoon salt

½ cup vinegar

1 medium onion, chopped

1 (15½-ounce) can dark red kidney beans, drained and rinsed

½ cup celery, chopped

1 green pepper, chopped

1. Cook frozen vegetables according to package directions. Cool.
2. For dressing: Combine sugar, flour, dry mustard, and salt. Add vinegar. Cook until clear, stirring constantly. Allow dressing to cool.
3. For salad: Combine cooked vegetables, celery, green

pepper, onion, and beans. Add dressing and toss to mix. Refrigerate several hours to blend the flavors. Stir beans into salad just before serving.

_____

Makes 8 servings.
Reprinted with permission from the Northarvest Bean Growers Association, www.northarvestbean.org.

• • •

Lemon Blueberry and Chicken Salad

¾ cup low-fat lemon yogurt

3 tablespoons reduced-calorie mayonnaise

1 teaspoon salt

2 cups fresh or frozen blueberries, divided (Reserve a few blueberries for garnish.)

2 cups cubed cooked chicken breasts

½ cup sliced green onions (scallions)

¾ cup diagonally sliced celery

½ cup diced sweet red bell pepper

1. In a medium bowl, combine yogurt, mayonnaise, and salt. Add blueberries, chicken, green onions, celery, and bell pepper; mix gently. Cover and refrigerate to let flavors blend, at least 30 minutes.
2. Serve over endive or other greens and garnished with reserved blueberries and lemon slices, if desired.

_____

Makes 4 servings.

Reprinted with permission from the U.S. Highbush Blueberry Council, www.blueberry.org.

◆ ◆ ◆

Blueberry Balsamic Vinegar

4 cups frozen, thawed, or fresh blueberries
1 quart balsamic vinegar
¼ cup sugar
Lime peel cut in strips from 1 lime (green part only)
1 (3-inch) cinnamon stick

1. In a large nonreactive saucepan, crush blueberries with a potato masher or back of a heavy spoon. Add vinegar, sugar, lime peel, and cinnamon stick; bring to a boil. Reduce heat and simmer, covered, for 20 minutes. Cool slightly and pour into a large bowl. Cover and refrigerate for 2 days to allow flavors to blend.
2. Place a wire mesh strainer over a large bowl. In batches, ladle blueberry mixture into strainer, pressing out as much liquid as possible. Discard solids.
3. Pour vinegar into clean glass bottles or jars; refrigerate, tightly covered, indefinitely. Use this in salad dressings or drizzled over grilled chicken or beef.

Makes 5½ cups.
Reprinted with permission from the U.S. Highbush Blueberry Council, www.blueberry.org

◆ ◆ ◆

Greek Potato Salad with Dried Tomatoes

**1 pound (3 medium) potatoes, uniform in size, cut into
¼-inch slices**

Lemon Dressing
¼ cup olive oil

¼ cup water

2½ tablespoons lemon juice

1 large clove garlic, pressed

**1 tablespoon chopped fresh oregano, or 1 teaspoon dried
oregano leaves**

1 teaspoon salt

½ teaspoon pepper

**1 cup (1½ ounces) dried tomato halves, halved with
kitchen shears**

1 cup sliced seedless cucumber

½ cup sliced red onion

1 cup crumbled feta cheese

½ cup Greek olives or pitted ripe olives

1. In a 2-quart saucepan over medium heat, cook potatoes, covered, in 2 inches boiling water until
   tender, about 12 minutes; drain and set aside.
2. Meanwhile, in a small bowl, cover tomatoes with
   boiling water; set aside 10 minutes while you whisk
   together olive oil, water, lemon juice, garlic, oregano, salt, and pepper for dressing.
3. Thoroughly drain tomatoes and pat dry with paper
   towels. Add potatoes, tomatoes, and cucumbers to
   bowl containing dressing; toss to coat. Mound potato mixture on plate. Arrange onion, cheese, and
   olives on top.

Makes 4 servings.
Reprinted with permission from the U.S. Potato Board,
www.potatohelp.com.

• • •

California Bulgur Salad with Lemon Mint Dressing

1 cup bulgur wheat

½ cup sliced mushrooms

2 tablespoons butter or margarine

2 cups chicken broth

¼ cup diagonally sliced green onions

Lemon Mint Dressing (recipe follows)

1 cup finely shredded red cabbage

2 to 3 (about 3 to 3½ ounce each) California kiwifruit, pared and sliced

1 (10- to 12-ounce) cooked chicken breast boned, skinned, and sliced

1. Sauté bulgur and mushrooms in butter until golden; add chicken broth, cover, and bring to boil. Reduce heat and simmer 15 minutes. Cool. Toss with green onions and ¼ cup Lemon Mint Dressing. Arrange bulgur, cabbage, and kiwifruit on plates with sliced chicken or fish; drizzle with remaining Lemon Mint Dressing.

2. Lemon Mint Dressing: Combine 6 tablespoons lemon juice, 2 tablespoons vegetable oil, and 4 teaspoons honey with 2 teaspoons each grated lemon peel and

Makes 4 servings.

fresh minced mint leaves (one teaspoon dried crushed mint can be substituted); mix well.

Makes about ¹/₂ cup.
Reprinted with permission from the California Kiwifruit Commission, www.kiwifruit.org

MAIN DISHES

Black Bean Burgers

Canola oil cooking spray

2 bunches finely chopped scallions, both white and green parts

1 red pepper, seeded and cut in ¹/₂-inch pieces

2 cloves garlic, finely chopped

1 (15-ounce) can black beans, drained and rinsed

1 cup cooked brown rice

Dash hot pepper sauce, or to taste

1 teaspoon cumin, or to taste

Salt and freshly ground black pepper to taste

1 large egg white, lightly beaten

¹/₂ cup whole-grain breadcrumbs

1. Heavily coat a medium skillet with canola oil cooking spray. Heat over medium-high heat until hot. Add scallions, red pepper, and garlic. Reduce heat to medium-low and sauté until very soft, about 5 minutes. Do not let vegetables brown.
2. Remove vegetables from heat and mix in beans and rice. Transfer to a food processor or blender and

process until mixture is coarsely chopped. Be careful not to overprocess.

3. Transfer mixture to a medium bowl. Season to taste with hot pepper sauce, cumin, salt, and pepper. Add egg white and mix in lightly with a fork until just blended. Mix in breadcrumbs with a fork until lightly blended. Form mixture into eight patties. (Patties will hold their shape better if refrigerated, covered, at least 30 minutes.)

4. When ready to sauté patties, lightly coat a skillet with cooking oil spray and heat over medium-high heat until hot. Add patties and sauté on both sides until nicely browned, about 4 minutes per side.

5. Serve plain or with lettuce and tomato on whole-grain buns.

_____

Makes 4 servings.

Reprinted with permission from the American Institute of Cancer Research, www.aicr.org

◆ ◆ ◆

Roasted Vegetable Wrap

1 small eggplant

3 teaspoons extra-virgin olive oil, divided

½ small bulb fennel, cut vertically in very thin slices

2 large mushrooms, thinly sliced

1 small zucchini, thinly sliced

1 small red pepper, seeded and cut in ¼-inch strips

8 thin slices red onion

8 to 12 whole garlic cloves, peeled

2 teaspoons minced fresh rosemary, or ½ teaspoon dried
and crushed

Salt and freshly ground pepper to taste

2 tablespoons soft, fresh goat cheese

1 (15-inch) piece soft cracker bread, or 2 (9-inch) wheat
tortillas

1. Preheat oven to 375 degrees. Spray two baking
   sheets with cooking spray.
2. Cut 4 slices vertically from eggplant, each ¼-inch
   thick. Set aside remaining eggplant for another use.
   Lay slices in one layer on one of the baking sheets.
   Pour ½ teaspoon olive oil on your palm and rub it
   over slices, turning so both sides are lightly coated.
   Do the same with fennel slices. Arrange both vegetables on the baking sheet. Roast until eggplant
   is tender, 12 to 15 minutes.
3. Meanwhile, toss mushrooms and zucchini in a bowl
   with 1 teaspoon olive oil. Arrange vegetables in one
   layer on second baking sheet. Roast until tender,
   about 10 minutes. Set aside.
4. Toss red pepper, onion, and garlic with remaining
   oil, rosemary, and, if desired, salt and pepper. Re-

using the baking sheet from eggplant, spread vegetables in one layer and roast until softened, about
15 minutes. Set aside.

5. To assemble wrap, thinly spread goat cheese on one
   side of bread to cover it completely. Arrange vegetables to cover two-thirds of bread, keeping
   cheese-only part at top. Start with eggplant,
   followed by fennel, red pepper mixture, and
   mushroom-zucchini mixture.

6. Roll up filled bread, jelly-roll fashion, starting at
   the bottom. To keep filling from pushing forward,
   keep pulling rolled part toward you. This also helps
   make a firm roll. Wrap and refrigerate from 4 to 48
   hours. To serve, cut into 2-inch slices.

Makes 4 servings.

Variation: Use whole-wheat pita bread in place of cracker
bread or tortillas.

Cooking for two: Make all the vegetables. Use the extra as a
side dish over the next day or two.

*Reprinted with permission from the American Institute of Cancer Re-
search, www.aicr.org.*

❖ ❖ ❖

Speedy Meatless Taco Filling

1 tablespoon canola oil

1 medium onion, chopped

2 garlic cloves, finely chopped

1 medium green bell pepper, seeded and chopped

1 teaspoon ground cumin

1 teaspoon dried oregano

½ cup fresh cilantro leaves, chopped

1 medium tomato, seeded and chopped

1 (12-ounce) package refrigerated or frozen soy crumbles

1½ cups prepared salsa

Dash of Tabasco sauce, or to taste (optional)

Salt and freshly ground black pepper to taste

1. In a large, nonstick skillet, heat oil until hot. Sauté onion, garlic, and green pepper until onion is translucent, about 4 minutes. Add cumin and oregano and mix until fragrant.
2. Add cilantro, tomato, soy crumbles, and salsa. Bring to a boil, reduce heat, and simmer 3 minutes. Season to taste with Tabasco sauce, salt, and pepper. Serve in taco shells, over cooked brown rice, or use to make nachos. Can store refrigerated up to 4 days.

_____

Makes 4 servings.
Reprinted with permission from the American Institute of Cancer Research, www.aicr.org.

• • •

White Chili

1 **pound dry navy beans**

1 **pound ground turkey, or 2 cups cooked, cubed turkey**

2 **(4-ounce) cans medium or hot green chili peppers, diced**

3 **tablespoons dry chicken bouillon**

2 **medium onions, chopped**

2 **teaspoons dry minced garlic**

2 **tablespoons whole cumin**

4 **ounces low-fat Monterey Jack cheese, shredded**

1. Soak beans using Preferred Hot Soak method: Add 10 cups of cold water to the beans. Bring the water to a boil, and boil for 3 minutes. Cover the pot, letting the beans soak for at least 4 hours. Then, drain and rinse soaked beans. Add fresh cold water to fully cover beans. Simmer the beans until they're tender. Brown ground turkey, drain, and discard fat. Combine in a slow cooker: beans and liquid, turkey, 1 can chili peppers, bouillon, onions, garlic, and cumin. Stir.
2. Cover and cook on low for several hours. Taste and add more chili peppers 1 tablespoon at a time if a hotter taste is desired. (Freeze leftover chili peppers.) Serve hot, topped with cheese.

Makes 12 servings.
Reprinted with permission from the Northarvest Bean Growers Association, www.northarvestbean.org.

SIDE DISHES

Red Potatoes with Kale

4 medium red potatoes

1 bunch kale

1 teaspoon toasted sesame oil

1 onion, thinly sliced

2 garlic cloves, minced

½ teaspoon black pepper

½ teaspoon paprika

5 teaspoons soy sauce

1. Scrub potatoes and cut into ½-inch cubes or wedges. Steam over boiling water until just tender when pierced with fork. Rinse with cold water, drain, and set aside.
2. Rinse kale and remove tough stems. Tear leaves into small pieces.
3. Heat oil in a large nonstick skillet and add onion and garlic. Sauté for 5 minutes.
4. Add cooked potatoes, pepper, and paprika, and continue cooking until potatoes begin to brown, about 5 minutes. Turn mixture gently as it cooks.
5. Spread kale leaves over top of potato mixture. Sprinkle with 2 tablespoons water and soy sauce. Cover and cook, turning occasionally, until kale is tender, about 7 minutes.

Makes 4 servings.
Reprinted with permission from the American Institute of Cancer Research, www.aicr.org.

• • •

Pineapple, Corn, and Mango Salsa

1 cup canned crushed pineapple (packed in its own juices), drained

½ medium mango, diced

½ cup frozen corn, thawed

½ cup chopped tomatoes

¼ cup minced parsley

3 tablespoons minced red onion

Salt, cayenne pepper, and cumin to taste

1. In medium bowl, mix pineapple, mango, corn, tomatoes, parsley, and onion. Season with salt, cayenne, and cumin to taste.
2. Serve over grilled fish, chicken, or tofu.

Makes 2½ cups.
Reprinted with permission from the American Institute of Cancer Research, www.aicr.org.

• • •

Risotto Primavera

3 cups fat-free, reduced-sodium chicken stock or broth

1 small green zucchini squash, cut in ½-inch dice

6 thin asparagus stalks, cut in ½-inch pieces, tips reserved

1 medium carrot, halved lengthwise and thinly sliced

1 tablespoon extra-virgin olive oil

¼ cup finely chopped Spanish onion

1 cup Arborio rice

2 teaspoons lemon juice, preferably fresh

1 small garlic clove, minced

½ cup fresh or frozen baby green peas

¼ cup chopped fresh flat-leaf parsley

1 tablespoon low-fat yogurt

2 tablespoons grated Parmigiano-Reggiano cheese

Salt and freshly ground black pepper to taste

1. Heat chicken stock to boiling. Set aside.
2. Place zucchini in a large bowl. Add asparagus and carrot and mix in.
3. Heat oil in a deep saucepan over medium-high heat. Add onion and sauté until translucent, about 2 minutes. Mix in rice until coated with oil and opaque, about 1 minute. Add lemon juice, stirring until rice is almost dry, less than 1 minute. Mix in garlic and half the chopped vegetables. Cook 1 minute.
4. Add hot broth, ½ cup at a time, stirring well after each addition. Cook, stirring continually, until rice is almost dry before adding more broth. When most of broth has been used and rice is almost done but has a hard core, about 15 to 18 minutes, add re-

maining vegetables and parsley. Add remaining broth and cook until rice is tender but still al dente (offering a slight resistance when bitten into, but not soft), about 3 to 4 minutes.

5. Remove pot from heat. Stir in yogurt and cheese. Season to taste with salt and pepper. Serve immediately.

Makes 5 servings.
Reprinted with permission from the American Institute of Cancer Research, www.aicr.org

♦ ♦ ♦

Grilled Potato Planks

3 tablespoons olive oil

1 clove garlic, minced

2 teaspoons finely chopped fresh rosemary leaves

½ teaspoon salt

1½ pounds (about 3 large) unpeeled baking potatoes, cut into ½ inch-thick slices

1. Preheat grill. Combine oil, garlic, rosemary, and salt in dish. Add potato slices and turn until well coated. Grill potatoes for 8 minutes or until soft. Turn and continue grilling 10 minutes longer or until cooked through.

2. Remove from grill and serve with your favorite grilled meals.

Makes 4 servings.
Reprinted with permission from the U.S. Potato Board, www.potatohelp.com.

• • •

Garlic Roasted Potatoes

3/4 pound (2 medium) potatoes, cut into wedges
1 tablespoon olive oil
2 small cloves garlic, finely chopped
1/2 teaspoon salt
1/4 teaspoon pepper
1 1/2 teaspoons finely chopped fresh parsley

1. Preheat oven 400 degrees. In a large bowl, toss together potatoes, oil, garlic, salt, and pepper until potatoes are well coated. Arrange potatoes in a single layer on a large baking sheet. Bake 1 hour or until browned and crisp, turning potatoes twice with a spatula during cooking.
2. Remove potatoes from oven and toss with parsley.

Makes 2 servings.
Reprinted with permission from the U.S. Potato Board, www.potatohelp.com.

• • •

Crunchy Seasoned Oven Fries

1 egg
3/4 cup cornflake crumbs

Italian Fries Seasoning
6 tablespoons grated Parmesan cheese
1 1/2 teaspoons Italian herb seasoning

Chili Fries Seasoning

1½ tablespoons chili powder
1½ teaspoons garlic salt
1⅓ pounds (4 medium) potatoes, cut into ½-inch-thick wedges

1. Heat oven to 375 degrees. Coat two baking sheets with vegetable cooking spray. Lightly beat egg in shallow bowl. In another shallow bowl, mix crumbs and seasoning blend of your choice. Dip potato wedges into egg, then coat completely with crumb mixture. Arrange in a single layer on baking sheets. Bake 20 minutes, then turn potatoes over and continue to bake 10 to 15 minutes longer, until potatoes are browned and crisp and insides are tender when tested with toothpick or fork.
2. Serve immediately, plain or with lemon or ketchup.

Makes 4 servings.
Reprinted with permission from the U.S. Potato Board, www.potatohelp.com

◆ ◆ ◆

Grilled Artichokes

4 large artichokes
¼ cup balsamic vinegar
¼ cup water
¼ cup soy sauce
1 tablespoon minced ginger
¼ cup olive oil

1. Slice artichoke tops off, crosswise. Trim stems.
2. Boil or steam artichokes until bottoms pierce easily or a petal pulls off easily.

3. Drain artichokes. Cool. Cut each artichoke in half lengthwise and scrape out fuzzy center and any purple-tipped petals.
4. Mix vinegar, water, soy sauce, ginger, and olive oil in a large plastic bag. Place artichokes in the bag and coat all sides of artichokes. For best flavor, marinate overnight in the refrigerator, but should marinate at least 1 hour.
5. Drain artichokes. Place cut side down on a grill over a solid bed of medium coals or gas grill on medium. Grill until lightly browned on the cut side, 5 to 7 minutes. Turn artichokes over and drizzle some of remaining marinade over artichokes. Grill until petal tips are lightly charred, 3 to 4 minutes more.
6. Serve hot or room temperature.

Makes 8 servings—¹/₂ artichoke each.
Reprinted with permission from the California Artichoke Advisory Board, www.artichokes.org.

• • •

Butternut Squash with Ginger

1 large butternut squash

1 tablespoon ginger root, freshly minced

¹/₄ cup unsweetened apple juice

Nutmeg, freshly ground

1. Preheat oven to 350 degrees.
2. Peel and seed squash and cut into ¹/₂-inch cubes. Put squash, ginger root, and apple juice into a lightly oiled baking dish.

3. Cover and bake for 50 to 60 minutes. Sprinkle with nutmeg just before serving.

***

Makes 4 servings.
Reprinted with permission from the Pioneer Valley Growers Association, www.pvga.net.

◆ ◆ ◆

Beet and Tomato Casserole

2½ cups canned beets, sliced

2½ cups canned tomatoes

½ cup grated cheese, any type

Salt and pepper to taste

2 cups breadcrumbs

1 tablespoon butter

1. Preheat oven to 350 degrees.
2. Put half the beets in the bottom of a greased baking dish. Add half the tomatoes then half the cheese in layers. Add salt and pepper, if desired. Add half the breadcrumbs. Dot with 1 tablespoon butter. Repeat with the rest of ingredients.
3. Cook for 20 minutes until brown.

***

Makes 6 servings.
Reprinted with permission from the Pioneer Valley Growers Association, www.pvga.net

DESSERTS

Red Berry Kissel

½ (20-ounce) bag whole, unsweetened frozen strawberries (about 10 ounces)

1 (10-ounce) package frozen sweetened raspberries

½ cup cranberry cocktail juice

3 tablespoons cornstarch

3 tablespoons cold water

½ teaspoon almond extract

1. Place frozen strawberries and raspberries in a deep
   saucepan. Add cranberry juice. Over medium-high
   heat, bring just to boil. Reduce heat and simmer
   until berries are very soft, about 20 minutes.
2. Pour berry mixture into fine sieve held over a bowl.
   With a wooden spoon, push berry pulp through the
   sieve. Scrape strained berries on the outside of the
   sieve into the bowl.
3. Rinse out and dry pot. Rinse four dessert dishes in
   cold water, but do not dry. Set aside.
4. Whisk berry mixture to combine pulp and liquid
   well. Return mixture to pot. Mix cornstarch and water in a small bowl. Stir mixture into berries. Add
   almond extract.
5. Over medium heat, cook mixture until translucent,
   stirring constantly. When mixture heavily coats
   spoon and thickens—about 1 to 2 minutes—remove from heat before it comes to a boil and pour
   into dessert dishes. When almost cool, refrigerate.
   To prevent surface skin from forming, cover bowls
   with plastic wrap, pressing it to touch the surface
   of pudding. Kissel can be made up to 2 days ahead.

6. Let kissel sit 20 minutes at room temperature before serving.

_____

Makes 4 servings.
Reprinted with permission from the American Institute of Can-
cer Research, www.aicr.org.

◆ ◆ ◆

Great Grilled Fruit Kebabs

2 tablespoons canola oil

2 tablespoons brown sugar

2 tablespoons fresh lemon juice

1 teaspoon cinnamon

**4 (1-inch) slices pineapple, canned or fresh, cut into
chunks**

2 apples, cored and cut into 1-inch pieces

2 pears, pitted and cut into 1-inch pieces

**2 peaches, nectarines, or plums (or a mix), pitted and cut
into 1-inch pieces**

2 bananas, peeled and cut into 1-inch pieces

1. In a small bowl, stir together oil, brown sugar,
lemon juice, and cinnamon until sugar is dissolved.
2. Thread pineapple, apples, pears, peaches, and bananas alternately onto each of eight skewers. Brush
kebabs with oil mixture and place skewers on bar-
becue grill. Turn frequently until fruit starts to
brown, about 6 to 8 minutes.

_____

Makes 8 servings.
Reprinted with permission from the American Institute of Can-
cer Research, www.aicr.org.

◆ ◆ ◆

Blueberry Orange Whirl

1 (12-ounce) package frozen blueberries, unthawed, or
2½ cups fresh blueberries

1 (8-ounce) container vanilla low-fat yogurt

½ cup orange juice

½ cup milk

1 teaspoon vanilla extract

1. In an electric blender, whirl blueberries, yogurt, orange juice, milk, and vanilla extract until smooth.
2. Serve immediately.

Makes 4 servings.
Reprinted with permission from the U.S. Highbush Blueberry Council, www.blueberry.org.

◆ ◆ ◆

Blueberry Granola Bars

½ cup honey

¼ cup firmly packed brown sugar

3 tablespoons vegetable oil

1½ teaspoons ground cinnamon

3½ cups quick-cooking oats

2 cups fresh blueberries

1. Preheat oven to 350 degrees. Lightly grease a 9 × 9-inch square baking pan. In a medium saucepan, combine honey, brown sugar, oil, and cinna-

mon. Bring to a boil, and boil for 2 minutes; do not stir. In a large mixing bowl, combine oats and blueberries. Stir in honey mixture until thoroughly blended. Spread into prepared pan, gently pressing mixture flat. Bake until lightly browned, about 40 minutes.

2. Cool completely in the pan on a wire rack. Cut into 1 ½ × 3-inch bars.

Makes 18 bars.
Reprinted with permission from the U.S. Highbush Blueberry Council, www.blueberry.org.

• • •

Kiwifruit Frozen Yogurt

2 California kiwifruit, peeled and coarsely chopped

1 tablespoon honey

1 pint frozen low-fat or nonfat vanilla yogurt, softened

1 to 2 drops green food coloring (optional)

1 (10-ounce) package frozen red raspberries in syrup, thawed

2 tablespoons triple sec or other orange liqueur

2 teaspoons cornstarch

3 California kiwifruit, ends trimmed and sliced lengthwise

Fresh mint leaves

Fresh or frozen whole raspberries (optional)

1. In a food processor or blender, purée 2 chopped kiwifruit; stir in honey. Place in freezer and freeze until slushy (about 45 minutes). In a stainless-steel bowl, quickly combine softened yogurt, kiwifruit

mixture, and food coloring (if using); refreeze in a bowl. With a small ice-cream scoop (about 2 tablespoons), form 12 balls and place on wax paper-lined tray; refreeze.

2. Meanwhile, to make sauce, in food processor or blender, purée thawed raspberries. Over a saucepan, strain berries through a fine sieve, pressing with the back of a spoon. Discard seeds. Stir in triple sec and cornstarch. Bring to boil, stirring constantly until slightly thickened. Cool; cover and chill. To assemble, spoon about 2 tablespoons sauce on each of six dessert plates or shallow bowls. Arrange kiwifruit slices and frozen yogurt balls on sauce. Garnish with mint leaves and whole raspberries.

Make 6 servings.

Reprinted with permission from the California Kiwifruit Commission, www.kiwifruit.com.

◆ ◆ ◆

Appendices

APPENDIX A

Glossary

ACRYLAMIDE. A carcinogen that forms as a result of chemical reactions that take place during baking or frying at high temperatures. It is found in high amounts in potato chips, corn chips, frozen french fries, and fast-food french fries.

ADVANCED GLYCATION END PRODUCTS (AGEs). Detrimental substances formed in the body when elevated blood sugar links up (or glycates) with proteins in the body. AGEs weaken bodily tissues, including blood vessels, and may set the stage for heart disease.

AEROBICS. Continuous-action exercise that can be performed within the body's ability to use and process oxygen. Examples include walking, jogging, running, cycling, swimming, and cross-country skiing.

ANTIOXIDANT. A special class of nutrients that fight "free radicals," a group of cells that damage otherwise healthy cells.

APPENDICITIS. An inflammation and infection of the appendix.

ATHEROSCLEROSIS. Narrowing and thinkening of the arteries caused by inflammation, or deposits of cholesterol, fats, and other substances.

CALORIES. Units that represent the amount of energy provided by food.

CANCER. A group of diseases characterized by the presence of cells that grow out of control.

CARBOHYDRATE COUNTING. A meal-planning system recommended for people with diabetes. This system estimates the number of carbohydrates in food and matches that amount to units of insulin.

CARBOHYDRATES. A food group that serves as a major energy source for the body. Derived mostly from sugar and starch, carbohydrates are broken down into glucose during digestion and are the main nutrient that elevates blood glucose levels.

CHOLESTEROL. A fatty substance found in some foods and manufactured by the body for many vital functions. Excess cholesterol and saturated fat can increase blood levels of cholesterol and can collect inside artery walls. This process contributes to heart disease.

COMPLEX CARBOHYDRATES. Carbohydrates (starches) made of multiple numbers of sugar molecules.

CONSTIPATION. A condition in which bowel movements occur less often than usual or consist of hard stools that are difficult to pass.

C-REACTIVE PROTEIN (CRP). A protein that increases with the amount of inflammation in your coronary arteries. High levels of CRP are now believed to be the strongest and most significant predictors of heart disease, heart attack, and stroke. CRP can be measured by medical testing.

CRUCIFEROUS VEGETABLES. Vegetables that contain indoles, compounds that seem to protect against cancer. Broccoli, cauliflower, cabbage, and watercress are cruciferous vegetables.

DEMENTIA. A condition in which a person gradually loses the ability to remember, think, reason, interact socially, and care for themself. It is not a disease, but rather a cluster of symptoms triggered by diseases or conditions that adversely affect the brain. Alzheimer's disease is one example of a dementia.

DIABETES. A disease in which the body cannot produce enough insulin or cannot use insulin in a normal way. This leads to high levels of glucose in the blood.

DIGESTION. The breakdown of foods by enzymes so that nutrients can be absorbed by the body.

DIVERTICULITIS. The development of inflammation and infection in one or more diverticuli, which are bulges in the inner lining of the colon.

DIVERTICULOSIS. The formation of bulges (diverticuli) in inner lining of the colon.

DUODENAL ULCER. A hole or break in the first part of the small intestine known as the duodenum.

ENERGY GELS. A type of highly concentrated carbohydrates with a puddinglike consistency that are packaged in single-serve pouches. Energy gels are designed for athletes and exercisers.

FATS. A food group that provides energy but is the most concentrated source of calories in the diet.

FATTY ACIDS. Components of either dietary fat or body fat.

FIBER. The nondigestible portion of plants that can lower fat and glucose absorption, assist in weight control, and promote a healthy digestive system.

FREE RADICALS. Cellular aberrations, formed when molecules somehow come up with an odd number of electrons. These cells destroy healthy cells by robbing them of oxygen, and this robbery weakens the immune system.

FRUCTOSE. A simple sugar found in fruit and fruit juices.

FRUCTOSE INTOLERANCE. A sensitivity to the fructose in fruit juices, sports drinks, or products containing high-fructose corn syrup, and sometimes to the natural fructose in fruit.

GALACTOSE. A simple sugar that is a part of lactose.

GALLSTONES. Solid crystal deposits, usually made up mostly of cholesterol, that form in the gallbladder, an organ that is involved in digestion.

GHRELIN. A hormone produced mostly by cells in your stomach that triggers your desire to eat.

GLUCAGON. A hormone produced by the pancreas that opposes the action of insulin and helps liberate fat from storage.

GLUCOSE. Blood sugar. It serves as a fuel for the body.

GLYCEMIC INDEX OF FOODS. A system of rating foods according to how fast they elevate blood glucose. Foods lower on the scale—low-glycemic index foods—are sometimes recommended in nutritional therapy for diabetes and weight control.

GLYCOGEN. Stored carbohydrates in the muscles and liver.

H. PYLORI. Bacterium that live in the mucous membranes lining the digestive tract that are the most common cause of duodenal ulcers.

HDL (HIGH-DENSITY LIPOPROTEIN). A type of cholesterol in the blood that has a protective effect against the buildup of plaque in the arteries.

HEMORRHOIDS. Swollen blood vessels in the anus, often the result of straining during a bowel movement.

HIGH-FIBER DIET. A food plan that supplies between 25 and 35 grams of fiber daily.

HIGH-FRUCTOSE CORN SYRUP. Made from corn starch, high-fructose corn syrup is a liquid comprised of roughly half fructose and half glucose and added to many processed foods, including soft drinks.

HYPERGLYCEMIA. Abnormally high levels of glucose in the blood.

HYPOGLYCEMIA. Low blood sugar.

INFLAMMATION. A bodily immune response that is triggered when the body is under attack from germs and other invaders.

INSOLUBLE FIBER. A type of fiber that supplies bulk to keep foods moving through the digestive system.

INSULIN. A hormone that decreases blood glucose levels by moving glucose into cells to be used for fuel. It is also involved in protein synthesis and fat formation.

INSULIN RESISTANCE. A condition in which cells do not respond to insulin properly.

INSULINLIKE GROWTH FACTORS. Chemicals in the body that arise with increased insulin production. When produced in excess, they might promote cancer by increasing abnormal cell growth.

IRRITABLE BOWEL SYNDROME. A condition characterized by alternating periods of diarrhea and constipation, often accompanied by cramping.

LACTOSE. The simple sugar found in milk.

LACTOSE INTOLERANCE. A sensitivity to the simple sugar lactose in milk. It is caused by the lack of sufficient lactase, the enzyme required to digest lactose.

LEPTIN. A hormone produced in the body that acts like an appetite suppressant.

LIPOPROTEIN LIPASE (LPL). An enzyme governing fat storage.

LOW-DENSITY LIPOPROTEINS (LDL). A type of cholesterol in the blood. High levels contribute to coronary heart disease.

MALTOSE. A simple sugar found in plants during the early stages of germination.

METABOLIC RATE. The speed at which your body burns calories.

METABOLIC SYNDROME (SYNDROME X). A cluster of symptoms that set the stage for type II diabetes and heart disease. These symptoms include glucose intolerance, central obesity, elevated blood fats, and high blood pressure.

METABOLISM. The physiological process that converts food to energy so the body can function.

MINERAL. A class of nutrients needed by the body for a wide range of enzymatic and metabolic functions.

MONOSACCHARIDE. A type of simple sugar constructed of a single molecule of glucose.

MONOUNSATURATED FAT. Fatty acids that lack two hydrogen atoms. Found in such foods as olive oil, olives, avocados, cashew nuts, and cold-water fish such as salmon, mackerel, halibut, and swordfish.

OBESITY. An excessive and abnormal amount of weight, usually 20 percent or more above a person's ideal weight. Obesity is a risk factor for heart disease, cancer, and type II diabetes.

PHOTOSYNTHESIS. A process in which the sun's energy is captured by chlorophyll, the green coloring in leaves, to turn water from the soil and carbon dioxide from the air into an energy-yielding sugar called glucose.

PHYTOCHEMICALS. A large group of health-bestowing chemicals found in plant foods.

POLYSACCHARIDE. Multiple number of sugar molecules linked together in a long chain. Complex carbohydrates (starches) are polysaccharides.

POLYUNSATURATED FAT. A fatty acid found in fish and in most vegetable oils.

PREBOTICS. A type of undigested carbohydrate technically known as "fructooligosaccharides," or FOS, for short. FOS become a "meal" for health-promoting bacteria such as acidophilus (known as a probiotic), believed to enhance healthy flora in the intestines, improve digestion, and prevent disease.

PROTEIN. A food group necessary for growth and repair of body tissues.

RIBOSE. A beneficial simple sugar that forms the carbohydrate backbone of DNA and RNA, the genetic material that controls cellular growth and reproduction, thus governing all life. Available as a supplement marketed to exercisers and athletes.

SATURATED FAT. A fatty acid that is solid at room temperature.

SIMPLE SUGARS. A type of carbohydrate that is constructed of either single or double molecules of glucose.

SOLUBLE FIBER. A type of fiber in grains, legumes, and carrots that has been shown to reduce cholesterol and slow the release of glucose into the bloodstream.

STARCH. A type of carbohydrate consisting of three or more glucose molecules. Most plant foods, including cereals, whole grains, pasta, fruits, and vegetables, are complex carbohydrates.

STRENGTH TRAINING. Any kind of weight-bearing activity in which your muscles are challenged to work harder each time they're exercised.

STROKE. Bleeding or lack of blood supply in the brain.

SUGAR. A form of carbohydrate that supplies calories and can elevate blood glucose levels.

SUGAR SUBSTITUTES. Sweeteners that can be used in place of sugar to reduce calories or control glucose levels. Substitutes include saccharin, aspartame, acesulfame-K, sugar alcohols, stevia (an herb), and tagatose.

TAGATOSE. A low-calorie natural sugar that has been recently approved by the FDA for use in foods, beverages, and other products.

TRIGLYCERIDES. Fats that circulate in the blood until they are deposited in fat cells. Elevated triglycerides (above 200) are a risk factor for heart disease.

TYPE I DIABETES. A form of diabetes that develops prior to age thirty but can occur at any age. It is caused by an immune system attack on the body's own beta cells. When these cells are destroyed, insulin can no longer be produced.

TYPE II DIABETES. A form of diabetes that occurs in people over age forty but can develop in younger people. With type II diabetes, the body does not use insulin properly.

UNSATURATED FAT. Fats that are liquid at room temperature.

VITAMINS. Organic substances found in food that perform many vital functions in the body.

APPENDIX B

References

A portion of the information in this book comes from medical research reports in both popular and scientific publications, professional textbooks and booklets, books, Internet sources, and computer searches of medical databases of research abstracts.

Chapter One: The Food Fuel

Brown, J. *The Science of Human Nutrition*. San Diego: Harcourt Brace Jovanovich, 1990.

Deutsch, R. M., *et al. Realities of Nutrition*. Palo Alto, CA: Bull Publishing Company, 1993.

Herbert, V., *et al. Total Nutrition*. New York: St. Martin's Press, 1995.

Kleiner, S. M. "Antioxidant Answers." *The Physician and Sportsmedicine*. 24:21–22, 1996.

Jequier, E. "Carbohydrates as a Source of Energy." *American Journal of Clinical Nutrition*. 59:682S–685S, 1994.

Chapter Two: Carbohydrate Scorecards

Begley, S. "Beyond Vitamins." *Newsweek,* April 25, 1994, pp. 44–49.

Blumenthal, D. "A Simple Guide to Complex Carbs." *FDA Consumer.* 23:13–17, 1989.

"Diet. The Glycemic Index." *Harvard Health Letter.* 24:7, 1999.

Foster-Powell, K., *et al.* "International Tables of Glycemic Index." *American Journal of Clinical Nutrition.* 62:871S–890S, 1995.

Frost, G. "The Relevance of the Glycemic Index to Our Understanding of Dietary Carbohydrate." *Diabetic Medicine.* 17:336–345, 2000.

Glycemic Index Research Institute. *The Complete Guide to Fat-Storing Carbohydrates.* Washington, DC: Glycemic Index Research Institute, 2000.

Kleiner, S. M. "Antioxidant Answers." *The Physician and Sportsmedicine.* 24:21–22, 1996.

Morris, K. L., *et al.* "Glycemic Index, Cardiovascular Disease, and Obesity." *Nutrition Review.* 57:273–276, 1999.

Chapter Three: Healthy Bites: The Twenty-five Super Carbs

"Gut Guard: Vitamin E Against Tumor-Friendly Damage." *Prevention,* February 1994, pp. 18–19.

"Vitamins, Carotenoids, and Phytochemicals." www.webmd.com, 1999.

Gebhardt, R. "Antioxidant and Protective Properties of Extracts from Leaves of the Artichoke (*Cynara scolymus L.*) Against Hydroperoxide-Induced Oxidative Stress in

Cultured Rat Hepatocytes." *Toxicology and Applied Pharmacology.* 144:279–286, 1997.

McCord, H. "Nature's Best Cholesterol Crunchers." *Prevention,* May 1, 1994, pp. 54–62.

Ness, A. R., *et al.* "Fruit and Vegetables, and Cardiovascular Disease: A Review." *International Journal of Epidemiology.* 26:1–13, 1997.

Segasothy, M., *et al.* "Vegetarian Diet: Panacea for Modern Lifestyle Diseases?" *Quarterly Journal of Medicine.* 92:531–544, 1999.

Chapter Four: Your Brain on Carbs

Blaun, R. "How to Eat Smart." *Psychology Today.* 29:34– 44, 1996.

Greenwood-Robinson, M. *20/20 Thinking.* New York: Avery Books, 2003.

Jeerkathil, T. J., *et al.* "Prevention of Strokes." *Current Atherosclerosis Reports.* 3:321–327, 2001.

Korol, D. L., *et al.* "Glucose, Memory, and Aging." *American Journal of Clinical Nutrition.* 67:746S–671S, 1998.

Trankina, M. "Choosing Foods to Modulate Moods." *The World & I.* 13:150, 1998.

Wurtman, J. J. "Carbohydrate Cravings: A Disorder of Food Intake and Mood." *Clinical Neuropharmacology.* 11:S139–145, 1988.

Wurtman, J. J. "Effect of Nutrient Intake on Premenstrual Depression." *American Journal of Obstetrics and Gynecology.* 161:1228–1234, 1989.

Wurtman, R. J. "Nutrients Affecting Brain Composition and Behavior." *Integrative Psychiatry.* 5:226–238, 1987.

Chapter Five: The Carb-Cancer Connection

American Institute for Cancer Research. "Food, Nutrition, and the Prevention of Cancer: A Global Perspective." www.aicr.org, 2002.

———. "Simple Steps to Prevent Cancer." www.aicr.org, 2002.

Associated Press. "Cancer Could Rise 50 Percent, U.S. Says." *Daily News*. April 4, 2003, p. B6.

Augustin, L. S., *et al.* "Dietary Glycemic Index and Glycemic Load, and Breast Cancer Risk: A Case-Controlled Study." *Annals of Oncology*. 12:1533–1538, 2001.

Berrino, F., *et al.* "Reducing Bioavailable Sex Hormones Through a Comprehensive Change in Diet: The Diet and Androgens (DIANA) Randomized Trial." *Cancer Epidemiology, Biomarkers & Prevention*. 10:25–33, 2001.

De Stefani, E., *et al.* "Dietary Sugar and Lung Cancer: A Case-Controlled Study in Uruguay." *Nutrition and Cancer*. 31:132–137, 1998.

Fox, M. C. "Control Carbs, Control Cancer." *Prevention*. January 1, 2003, p. 119.

Franceschi, S., *et al.* "Dietary Glycemic Load and Colorectal Cancer Risk." *Annals of Oncology*. 12:173–178, 2001.

Michaud, D. S., *et al.* "Dietary Sugar, Glycemic Load, and Pancreatic Cancer Risk in a Prospective Study." *Journal of the National Cancer Institute*. 94:1293–1300, 2002.

Nijveldt, R. J. "Flavonoids: A Review of Probable Mechanisms of Action and Potential Applications." *American Journal of Clinical Nutrition*. 74:418–425, 2001.

Slattery, M. I., *et al.* "Dietary Sugar and Colon Cancer." *Cancer Epidemiology, Biomarkers & Prevention.* 6:677–685, 1997.

Slavin, J. I., *et al.* "Plausible Mechanisms for the Protectiveness of Whole Grains." *American Journal of Clinical Nutrition.* 70:459S–463S, 1999.

Steinmetz, K. A., *et al.* "Vegetables, Fruit, and Cancer Prevention: A Review." *Journal of the American Dietetic Association.* 96:1027–1039, 1996.

Tipton, M., "Selenium May Cut the Risk of Prostate Cancer." *Medical Update.* 22:3, 1998.

Chapter Six: The Diabetes Defense

American Diabetes Association. "Diabetes Info." www.diabetes.org, 2001.

———. "Evidence-Based Nutrition Principles and Recommendations for the Treatment and Prevention of Diabetes and Related Complications." *Diabetes Care.* 26:S51–S61, 2003.

———. "Nutrition Guide for People with Diabetes." www.diabetes.org, 2003.

Arcement, P. S. "Carbohydrate Counting in Diabetes Meal Planning." *Home Healthcare Nurse.* 17:425–428, 1999.

Benedict, M. "Carbohydrate Counting. Tips for Simplifying Diabetes Eduction." *Health Care Food & Nutrition Focus.* 16:6–9, 1999.

Daly, A., *et al.* "Carbohydrate Counting: Getting Started." Chicago, IL: American Dietetics Association, 1995.

Greenwood-Robinson, M. *Control Diabetes in 6 Easy Steps.* New York: St. Martin's Press, 2002.

Chapter Seven: Digestive Health

Black, J. "Acute Appendicitis in Japanese Soldiers in Burma: Support for the "Fibre" Theory." *Gut.* 51:297, 2002.

Brown, E. W. "50,000 Unnecessary Appendectomies a Year—and How to Prevent Them." *Medical Update.* 20:4, 1997.

Carson-Dewitt, R. S. "Diverticulosis and Diverticulitis." *Gale Encyclopedia of Medicine.* www.findarticles.com, 1999.

Dosh, S. A. "Evaluation and Treatment of Constipation." *Journal of Family Practice.* www.findarticles.com, June 2002.

Flagg, S., *et al.* "Gut Protection." *Prevention.* January 1, 1997, pp. 31–32.

Haggerty, M. "Constipation." *Gale Encyclopedia of Medicine.* www.findarticles.com, 1999.

Marlatt, J., *et al.* "Position of the American Dietetic Association: Health Implications of Dietary Fiber." *Journal of the American Dietetic Association.* 102:993–1000, 2002.

Murray, M. T. *Encyclopedia of Nutritional Supplements.* Rocklin, Cal.: Prima Publishing, 1996.

Ortega, R. M., *et al.* "Differences in Diet and Food Habits Between Patients with Gallstones and Controls." *Journal of the American College of Nutrition.* 16:88–95, 1997.

Paradox. P. "Gallstones." *Gale Encyclopedia of Alternative Medicine.* www.findarticles.com, 2001.

Swade, S. "Ease Gut Reactions." *Prevention.* February 1, 1995, pp. 78–80.

Todoroki I., *et al.* "Cholecystectomy and the Risk of Colon Cancer." *American Journal of Gastroenterology.* 94:41–46, 1999.

Trautwein, E. A. "Dietetic Influences on the Formation and Prevention of Cholesterol Gallstones." *Zeitschrift für Ernahrungswissenschaft.* 33:2–15, 1994.

Walker, A. R., *et al.* "What Causes Appendicitis?" *Journal Clinical Gastroenterology.* 12:127–129, 1990.

Weil, A. "Warning: 11 Medical Practices to Avoid." *East West Natural Health.* 22:58–63, 1992.

Wolnik, L., and H. Bauer. "Epidemiology of Ovarian Cancer." *Onkologie.* 2:96–101, 1979.

Chapter Eight: Heart-Healthy Carbs

Fallon, S., *et al.* "Diet and Heart Disease: Not What You Think." *Consumers' Research Magazine.* July 1, 1996, pp. 15–19.

Gee, S. "The AGEing Process (Advanced Glycation End Products)." *Diabetes Forecast.* 51:72–74, 1998.

Howard, B. V., *et al.* "Sugar and Cardiovascular Disease." *Circulation.* 106:523–527, 2002.

Hunter, B. T. "Confusing Consumers About Sugar Intake." *Consumers' Research Magazine.* January 1, 1995, pp. 14–17.

"Inflammation and Heart Disease." *Medical Update.* January 1, 2002, p. 6.

Katan, M. B. "Are There Good and Bad Carbohydrates for HDL Cholesterol?" *The Lancet.* 353:1029–1030, 1999.

Lemonick, M. "Lean and Hungrier Is a Recently Discovered Hormone." *Time.* June 3, 2002. p. 54.

Ness, A. R., *et al.* "Fruit and Vegetables, and Cardiovascular Disease: A Review." *International Journal of Epidemiology.* 26:1–13, 1997.

Park, A. "Beyond Cholesterol: Inflammation Is Emerging as a Major Risk Factor—and Not Just in Heart Disease." *Time.* November 25, 2002, p. 75.

Squires, S. "Sweet but Not So Innocent." *The Washington Post.* March 11, 2003, p. F01.

Chapter Nine: Carbs and Weight Control: The Good-Carb Diet

Ammon, P. K. "Individualizing the Approach to Treating Obesity." *Nurse Practitioner.* 24:27–31, 36–38, 1999.

Auchmutey, J. "Sugar Nation." *The Atlanta Journal-Constitution.* November 17, 2002, p. A1.

Burton-Freeman, B. "Dietary Fiber and Energy Regulation." *Journal of Nutrition.* 130:272S–275S, 2002.

Howarth, N. C., *et al.* "Dietary Fiber and Weight Regulation." *Nutrition Reviews.* 59:129–139, 2001.

Kersten, S. "Mechanisms of Nutritional and Hormonal Regulation of Lipogenesis." *EMBO Reports.* 282–286, 2001.

Ludwig, D. S. "Dietary Glycemic Index and Obesity." *Journal of Nutrition.* 130:280S–283S, 2000.

Roberts, S. B., *et al.* "The Influence of Dietary Composition on Energy Intake and Body Weight." *Journal of the American College of Nutrition.* 21:140S–145S, 2002.

Chapter Ten: Carb Power for Exercisers and Athletes

Akermark, C., *et al.* "Diet and Muscle Glycogen Concentration in Relation to Physical Performance in Swedish Elite Ice Hockey Players." *International Journal of Sports Nutrition.* 6:272–284, 1996.

Burke, L. M. "Nutrition for Post-Exercise Recovery." *International Journal of Sports Nutrition.* 1:214–224, 1997.

Chandler R. M., *et al.* "Dietary Supplements Affect the Anabolic Hormones After Weight-Training Exercise." *Journal of Applied Physiology.* 76:839–45, 1994.

Coyle, E. F. "Timing and Method of Increased Carbohydrate Intake to Cope with Heavy Training, Competition and Recovery." *Journal of Sports Sciences.* 9:29–51, 1991.

"How Do Sports Drinks Work?" Barrington, IL: The Gatorade Company, 2000.

Ivy, J. L. "Glycogen Resynthesis After Exercise: Effect of Carbohydrate Intake." *International Journal of Sports Medicine.* 19:S142–S145, 1998.

———. "Role of Carbohydrate in Physical Activity." *Clinics in Sports Medicine.* 18:469–484, 1999.

Kleiner, S. *Power Eating.* Champaign, IL: Human Kinetics, 1998.

Chapter Eleven: Your Smart-Carb Strategy

American Cancer Society. "ACS Nutrition Guidelines." www.cancer.org, 2003.

About the Author

Maggie Greenwood-Robinson, Ph.D., is one of the country's top health and medical authors. She is the author of *Good Fat vs. Bad Fat, The Bikini Diet, Foods That Combat Cancer, 20/20 Thinking, Control Diabetes in 6 Easy Steps, The Bone Density Test, Hair Savers for Women: A Complete Guide to Preventing and Treating Hair Loss, The Cellulite Breakthrough, Natural Weight Loss Miracles, Kava Kava: The Ultimate Guide to Nature's Anti-Stress Herb*, and *21 Days to Better Fitness*. She is also the coauthor of nine other fitness books, including the national bestseller *Lean Bodies, Lean Bodies Total Fitness, High Performance Nutrition, Power Eating*, and *50 Workout Secrets*.

Her articles have appeared in *Let's Live, Physical Magazine, Great Life, Shape* magazine, *Christian Single Magazine, Women's Sports and Fitness, Working Woman, Muscle and Fitness, Female Bodybuilding and Fitness*, and many other publications. She is a member of the Advisory Board of *Physical Magazine*. In addition, she has a doctorate in nutritional counseling.

Stay Healthy and Fit

The Fat to Muscle Diet
by Victoria Zak, Chris Carlin, M.S., R.D., and
Peter Vash, M.D., M.P.H.
0-425-11060-5

Win the Fat War
by Anne Alexander
0-425-18061-1

Win the Cholestral War
by Holly McCord, R.D.
0-425-18819-1

Botox
by Ron M. Shelton, M.D., with Terry Malloy
0-425-18917-1

Good Fat vs. Bad Fat
by Maggie Greenwood-Robinson, Ph. D.
0-425-18427-7

The Bikini Diet
by Maggie Greenwood-Robinson, Ph.D.
0-425-19078-1

Liposuction
by Ron M. Shelton, M.D., and Terry Malloy
0-425-19385-3